D1595737

Management of Heart and Lung
Transplant Patients

Management of Heart and Lung Transplant Patients

Edited by

PETER M SCHOFIELD
*Consultant Cardiologist and
Clinical Director of Cardiac Services,
Papworth Hospital,
Cambridge, UK*

and

PAUL A CORRIS
*Consultant Physician and Reader in Thoracic Medicine,
Freeman Hospital,
Newcastle upon Tyne, UK*

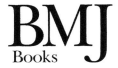

First published in 1998
by BMJ Books, BMA House, Tavistock Square,
London WC1H 9JR

British Library Cataloguing in Publication Data

A catalogue record for this book is available from the British Library

ISBN 0-7279-1365-4

Typeset by Apek Typesetters, Nailsea, Bristol
Printed and bound by Latimer Trend, Plymouth.

Contents

Contributors

Shinji Akamine
Consultant Surgeon
First Department of Surgery
Nagasaki School of Medicine
Japan

M B Anderson
Fellow in Cardiothoracic Surgery
Papworth Hospital
Cambridge

Peter C Braidley
Senior Surgical Transplant Fellow
Papworth Hospital,
Cambridge

N R B Cary
Consultant Histopathologist,
Papworth Hospital,
Cambridge

P A Corris
Consultant Physician and Reader in Thoracic Medicine,
Freeman Hospital,
Newcastle upon Tyne

J H Dark
Consultant Cardiothoracic Surgeon,
Freeman Hospital,
Newcastle upon Tyne

J J Egan
Consultant Respiratory Physician and Honorary Clinical Lecturer,
North West Lung Research Centre,
Wythenshawe Hospital,
Manchester

A El Gamel
Specialist Registrar
Cardiothoracic Transplant Centre,
Wythenshawe Hospital,
Manchester

Kate Gould
Consultant Microbiologist
Freeman Hospital,
Newcastle upon Tyne

Tim Higenbottam
Professor of Respiratory Medicine,
University of Sheffield Medical School

Stephen Large
Consultant Cardiac Surgeon,
Papworth Hospital,
Cambridge

Janet M McComb
Consultant Cardiologist
Freeman Hospital,
Newcastle upon Tyne

Jayan Parameshwar
Consultant Transplant Cardiologist
The Transplant Unit,
Papworth Hospital,
Cambridge

Peter M Schofield
Consultant Cardiologist and Clinical Director of Cardiac Services
Papworth Hospital
Cambridge

Susan Stewart
Consultant Histopathologist
Papworth Hospital,
Cambridge

John Wallwork
Consultant Cardiothoracic Surgeon and
Director of Transplantation
Papworth Hospital,
Cambridge

Foreword

This is an excellent book and the editors are to be congratulated for covering the whole field of heart and lung transplantation in an informative and authoritative way. The contributions are from four British transplant centres and are gratifyingly up to date which is important in a subject that has developed so rapidly in recent years.

In this respect it is interesting to reflect that after the failure of the first three heart transplants in London between 1968 and 1970, the Department of Health placed a moratorium on further clinical transplants and this prevailed until 1979 when first Papworth and then a year later Harefield began planned programmes. At that time there was considerable scepticism amongst the public and large sections of the medical profession as to the value and wisdom of pursuing what seemed to many an expensive procedure with little likelihood of success. However, the meticulous evaluation of the costs and benefits of the two programmes at Papworth and Harefield by Buxton and colleagues[1] led to government approval and supraregional designation of the service with appropriate funding and designation of a controlled number of new centres as these became needed. This became the envy of transplant workers in other countries, where lack of any such control often led to the establishment of many small centres with insufficient caseloads to build the necessary experience on.

The authors of this book suffered no such disadvantage and the chapters which follow reflect the best of current practice in all aspects of the management of heart and lung transplant patients. Although it would be invidious to identify individual contributions in a work of such general excellence, I found the two chapters on the general management of the lung transplant recipient and the histopathology of heart and lung transplantation to be particularly informative. However, the whole book should be of interest not only to trainees and specialists in this field but also to cardiologists, chest physicians and the many general physicians who are increasingly becoming involved in the management of this interesting group of patients.

Sir Terence English KBE DL FRCS

Reference

1 Buxton M, Acheson R M, Caine N, Gibson S, O'Brien B. *Costs and benefits of the heart transplant programmes at Harefield and Papworth Hospitals.* London. HMSO, 1985.

1 Identification of the suitable heart transplant recipient

Peter M Schofield

Introduction

The prognosis of patients with endstage cardiac failure is poor. During the last 20 years, cardiac transplantation has developed from an experimental procedure to an established therapeutic option for the treatment of patients with advanced myocardial disease.

There have been various developments which have led to the current success of heart transplantation: the establishment of appropriate surgical techniques, the development of methods to detect allograft rejection prior to the occurrence of symptoms, and the introduction of cyclosporin-based immunosuppression.

In the early 1960s Shumway and his colleagues developed the current technique for orthotopic cardiac transplantation. Although the operation could be performed successfully, long-term survival was precluded by the lack of potent and specific immunosuppressive agents and the inability to diagnose rejection at an early stage. In the 1970s right ventricular biopsy was introduced. This enabled the diagnosis of milder forms of allograft rejection and subsequent treatment resulted in an improvement of patient survival. In the 1980s, with the introduction of cyclosporin-based immunosuppression, there was a further marked improvement in patient survival. This led to the rapid expansion of the number of transplant centres worldwide.

There was a progressive increase in the number of patients undergoing cardiac transplantation during the 1980s. More recently, a plateau has been reached in terms of activity due to the limited availability of donor organs (Figure 1.1). It has been estimated that patients undergoing cardiac transplantation represent only a small proportion of the total population of patients with endstage cardiac failure who could potentially benefit from this treatment option.[1] How should we decide which patients should receive

1

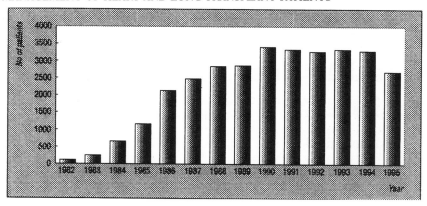

Fig 1.1 The number of transplants carried out worldwide each year between 1982 and 1995.

the available organs? On the basis of clinical findings and the results of invasive and non-invasive investigations, it is usually obvious which patients are severely disabled by left or right ventricular failure or both. The first question to ask is: "Is it likely that this patient would return to normal or near-normal if their heart was replaced?". Clearly the procedure is not appropriate if the patient has severe coexisting cerebrovascular disease, peripheral vascular disease, pulmonary disease or renal disease. In some patients, however, combined organ transplantation (e.g. heart and kidney) may be feasible. Patients accepted for cardiac transplantation should be well motivated and able to cope with immunosuppressive treatment after operation and also the inconvenience of repeated endomyocardial biopsy, particularly in the early postoperative period.

There has been a progressive improvement in patient survival following cardiac transplantation. In the early 1970s, one-year survival was only about 40%; by the early 1980s, it had increased to at least 60% following the more routine use of endomyocardial biopsy. In the 1990s the one-year survival is between 80% and 90% at most major centres.[2] Worldwide data from the International Society for Heart and Lung Transplantation (ISHLT) indicate five-year survival rates of 75%. As long-term survival has improved, additional problems have been encountered. These include the development of occlusive disease in the coronary arteries of the trans-planted heart and the adverse effects associated with long-term immunosuppressive therapy. In recent years, there has been a marked increase in the use of angiotensin-converting enzyme inhibitors in the treatment of endstage cardiac failure. None-the-less, the survival rate at 12 months in a group treated with enalapril was only around 50%.[3] Clearly, the quality of life as well as its duration must be considered. This has been shown to be substantially improved by cardiac transplantation, which has a good cost:benefit ratio.[4]

Indications

Most patients undergoing cardiac transplantation in our unit have heart failure refractory to medical treatment associated with either coronary artery disease (53%) or dilated cardiomyopathy (44%). This resembles the experience worldwide — 40% and 51% respectively. The timing of cardiac transplantation may be difficult in some patients. The symptoms of cardiac decompensation in those with coronary artery disease often remains stable, unless there is an event causing further myocardial damage and sudden death is a continuing risk. In contrast, the condition of those with dilated cardiomyopathy can deteriorate quite rapidly or in some cases improve, making their assessment for transplantation and the timing of surgery even more difficult. Therefore, careful and frequent follow-up is required for each patient.

The remaining group of patients undergoing cardiac transplantation (in our series 3% of the total population) includes those with other types of cardiomyopathy (for example, hypertrophic or restrictive), endstage valve disease, severe angina caused by coronary artery disease which is not amenable to revascularisation, and patients with ventricular tachyar-rhythmias which are refractory to other forms of treatment (Figure 1.2). Occasionally, therefore, it may be appropriate to give a cardiac transplant to a patient who is severely limited by angina rather than the symptoms of cardiac failure, if they are unsuitable for revascularisation procedures.

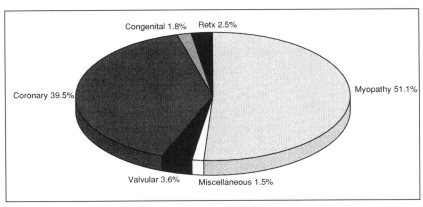

Fig 1.2   The indications for heart transplantation worldwide in adults (myopathy, cardiomyopathy; coronary, coronary artery disease; valvular, valvular heart disease; RETX, retransplantation; congenital, congenital heart disease; Misc., miscellaneous).

Patients with malignant ventricular tachyarrhythmias, many of whom have advanced left ventricular dysfunction, are an interesting group. Transplantation should be considered in those who are severely restricted by symptoms of cardiac failure. In other patients, drug treatment or implantation of a cardioverter-defibrillator may be appropriate. Antiarrhythmic surgery with intraoperative mapping and possibly concomitant bypass surgery is a further option.

In view of the limited availability of donor organs, one should always consider other treatment options. About 6% of patients referred with a view to cardiac transplantation, in our experience, are suitable for "conventional" cardiac surgery. This may involve a left ventricular aneurysmectomy or mitral valve surgery, with or without myocardial revascularisation. Clearly, cardiac catheterisation will establish the cause of cardiac failure and will determine whether any conventional treatment would be of benefit.

The selection of appropriate patients for cardiac transplantation is a major factor in determining the long-term survival. The selection of patients who are "too sick" for transplantation is a disservice, both to the patient and to others on the waiting list, since the chances of success are low. Conversely, we should not transplant patients who are doing well on medical therapy. Patients most likely to do well following cardiac transplantation are young, previously active individuals with stable symptoms from endstage heart disease who have single-organ failure. In an individual patient, it is not easy to determine the exact short-term prognosis or projected survival on medical treatment. In each case, a clinical judgement has to be made based on knowledge of prognostic indicators and an awareness of the various contraindications to cardiac transplantation.

Issues for consideration

Many of the "exclusion criteria" for cardiac transplantation have been modified over time as survival has improved and experience has been gained. In many transplant centres, insulin-dependent diabetics are now routinely transplanted and patients with previously "cured" malignant disease are offered this treatment option. For each patient, however, it is important to consider various issues which may be a relative or absolute contraindication to cardiac transplantation.

Age

The mean age of heart transplant recipients has increased slowly in recent years. Some studies have demonstrated no difference in early or late survival in patients transplanted over the age of 50 and have not detected the incidence of rejection or infection to be higher in the older transplant population.[5] Biological age as well as chronological age should be considered. Whilst survival may be comparable, morbidity may be significantly higher in older patients – for example, cataracts, weight gain, proximal muscle weakness, osteoporosis with compression fractures and diabetes mellitus related to chronic steroid administration.[6]

The age range for recipients of cardiac transplants worldwide is one day to 78 years[2] and, in our own units, six to 63 years. Although many units do not have absolute chronological limits, we tend to consider around 55 years for patients with coronary artery disease and around 60 years for those with dilated cardiomyopathy as a guide to the upper age limit. The differential is because we have found vascular complications in the early postoperative period, particularly cerebrovascular events and gastrointestinal ischaemia, to be more common in the older patient with underlying coronary artery disease.

The role of heart transplantation in neonates and infants continues to evolve. Neonatal transplantation has become established in the treatment of hypoplastic left heart syndrome and a variety of other complex congenital heart diseases. The use of cyclosporin and azathioprine for immunosuppression, with absent or minimal steroid usage, has minimised growth retardation and other complications. However, the long-term results of transplantation in patients under five years of age remain uncertain.

Pulmonary vascular resistance

Severe pulmonary hypertension remains an absolute contraindication to orthotopic cardiac transplantation. Many patients with chronic left-sided heart failure develop elevation of the mean pulmonary artery pressure and pulmonary vascular resistance (PVR). Those with a high, fixed PVR should not be considered for orthotopic transplantation, since the non-hypertrophied right ventricle of the donor heart cannot adapt to the acute afterload demands in the immediate postoperative period. The high postoperative mortality is due to acute right heart failure.

The risk of mortality within the first 30 days of cardiac transplantation increases in a continuous manner with increasing PVR, rather than being defined sharply at any specific level.[8] Some units would consider the presence of a fixed PVR in excess of 5–6 Wood units to be an absolute contraindication to orthotopic cardiac transplantation. Many centres now believe that the transpulmonary gradient (TPG), the difference between mean pulmonary artery pressure and the mean pulmonary capillary wedge pressure, is a better predictor of the risk of acute right ventricular failure following surgery.[9] We believe that a TPG of more than 15 mmHg which is fixed, precludes orthotopic cardiac transplantation while others use a value of 12 mmHg. Patients with a fixed TPG of more than 12 mmHg have a

5

5–7-fold increase in mortality at six months following surgery.[9] Some patients have a high TPG and/or high PVR which has a degree of reversibility. If the values fall to "acceptable levels" during the administration of oxygen, the intravenous infusion of sodium nitroprusside or prostaglandin, then they may have an acceptable risk for orthotopic transplantation although this may be higher than average.

Pulmonary vascular resistance measurements can change with time, so that patients on the waiting list for surgery should be reassessed every 4–6 months, particularly those whose levels are towards the upper end of the acceptable range. In many centres, patients who have a borderline PVR or TPG are transplanted using an "oversized" donor heart (i.e. a recipient-to-donor mismatch of greater than 20% of body weight). An alternative practice is the "domino" procedure in which the heart from a heart-lung recipient (for example, one who has primary pulmonary hypertension or cystic fibrosis), which has a prestressed right ventricle is used as the donor organ. Although in theory this approach seems logical, experience is too limited to make definitive conclusions. For those patients who have a high and fixed TPG and/or PVR and who are considered unsuitable for orthoptic cardiac transplantation, then heart-lung transplantation may be a consideration.

Other medical problems

Cardiac transplantation may not be an appropriate treatment for patients who have advanced disease in other systems. There is little point in offering surgery to patients who have advanced pulmonary disease. Many patients undergoing cardiac transplantation, however, will have some pulmonary disease but clinical judgement needs to be exercised in each individual patient.

Patients with chronic renal failure, with a creatinine clearance of < 30 ml/min, are usually not considered for cardiac transplantation. Similarly, patients with chronic hepatitis not explained by advanced right heart failure or cirrhosis are unsuitable. In some such cases, however, the results of combined organ transplantation can be extremely good – for example, heart and kidney or heart and liver. Once again, careful selection of patients and collaboration with the other appropriate transplant unit are vital to a successful outcome.

Some patients, in particular those with underlying coronary artery disease, may have associated peripheral vascular disease or cerebrovascular disease. If this is advanced and produces significant limitation of the patient's exercise capacity, there seems little point in undertaking cardiac transplantation. Patients who have made a good functional recovery after a cerebrovascular ischaemic event associated with thromboembolism from the left ventricle, usually in the setting of a dilated cardiomyopathy, but who do not have significant carotid artery disease may in fact do well with cardiac transplantation.

Patients with chronic hepatitis B antigen positivity are not usually considered for heart transplantation, since they are at risk of progressive hepatic dysfunction and cirrhosis, which is accelerated by chronic immunosuppression, particularly in the presence of "core" antigen. The presence of active systemic infection and HIV positivity also preclude cardiac transplantation.

Patients with a previous history of malignant disease may be referred for consideration for cardiac transplantation. They may have had Hodgkin's disease or childhood leukaemia and developed cardiomyopathy as a result of high-dose adriamycin therapy. Other patients who have had breast, bowel or lung cancer and who have been disease-free for over five years may be considered. It would appear that such patients experience identical survival to more traditional transplant recipients, providing that a complete staging evaluation (including chest and abdominal CT scanning) and other surveillance studies have shown freedom from disease for at least five years.[10] To date, there have been no reports of a higher incidence of second malignancies or recurrence of primary tumour in this group of patients.

Diabetes mellitus

In the past, patients with diabetes mellitus were not considered for cardiac transplantation because the risks of infection and accelerated coronary artery disease in the transplanted heart were considered too great. More recently, however, patients with insulin-dependent diabetes have undergone cardiac transplantation without a significant increase in infection, allograft rejection or two-year mortality.[7] It is important to ensure that diabetic patients are free of complications such as advanced proliferative retinopathy, severe peripheral neuropathy, peripheral or cerebrovascular atherosclerotic disease and chronic infections or ulceration of the feet. In selected patients, results comparable to non-diabetics can be achieved.

Social support/psychological stability

Patients undergoing cardiac transplantation have to endure far more investigation and treatment than patients following routine cardiac surgery, particularly in the early postoperative period. This includes repeated invasive assessment for rejection with right ventricular biopsy and careful monitoring for infection. Patients therefore require appropriate social support from family and/or friends. They must also have the ability to cope when complications occur in the postoperative period, usually allograft rejection or infections requiring treatment. It is important to explain these

---

Box 1.1 *Absolute contraindications to cardiac transplantation*

- Fixed and high pulmonary vascular resistance (PVR) and/or transpulmonary gradient (TPG)
- Active systemic infection
- Active peptic ulcer disease
- HIV positive or hepatitis B positive
- Recent malignant disease
- Life expectancy markedly compromised by other systemic disease
- Psychological instability/unable to comply with immunosuppressive regime

---

issues to patients in detail before listing them for cardiac transplantation. They should also be able to comply with a fairly complicated regime of medication postoperatively. Non-compliance with the immunosuppressive treatment is usually fatal.

It is possible, therefore, to identify some absolute and relative contra-indications to cardiac transplantation (Boxes 1.1 and 1.2), as well as the accepted and probable indications (Box 1.3).

The assessment of patients

In view of the nature of cardiac transplantation and the care required postoperatively, the detailed assessment of patients preoperatively is even more important than with conventional cardiac surgery. Patients are usually admitted to hospital in most centres for a period of assessment; this serves to determine the patient's suitability for cardiac transplantation as well as being a period of education for the patient and their family/friends. It is important to point out clearly the potential benefits and risks involved with cardiac transplantation and the patient must be actively involved in the final

---

Box 1.2 *Relative contraindications to cardiac transplantation*

- Age more than 60 years
- "Borderline" pulmonary vacular resistance (PVR) or transpulmonary gradient (TPG)
- Recent pulmonary embolism or infection
- Significant peripheral vascular disease or cerebrovascular disease
- Advanced renal, hepatic or pulmonary dysfunction*
- Diabetes mellitus with evidence of end-organ disease

* Unless combined organ transplantation is a feasible option.

Box 1.3 *Indications for cardiac transplantation*

Accepted
- $VO_2max < 10$ ml/kg/min
- Severe myocardial ischaemia not amenable to revascularisation which markedly limits activity
- Recurrent symptomatic ventricular arrhythmias refractory to all other therapeutic options

Probable
- $VO_2max < 14$ ml/kg/min and major limitation of the patient's activities
- Symptomatic cardiac failure with instability of fluid balance and renal function

Inadequate
- Left ventricular ejection fraction < 20%
- History of ventricular arrhythmias
- History of functional class III or IV heart failure

---

decision. The assessment period also enabled patients to meet other health-care professionals who will be involved in their postoperative care (including nurses and physiotherapists) as well as patients who have already undergone cardiac transplantation.

At the time of assessment, the following investigations should be considered (some of these will already have been carried out by the referring physician):

- routine haematology, including full blood count;
- routine biochemistry, including urea and electrolytes and liver function tests;
- hepatitis B status and HIV status;
- screen for infection, including midstream urine specimen and nasal swab;
- 24-h urine collection for creatinine clearance;
- electrocardiogram and chest radiograph;
- echocardiography and Doppler assessment (chamber size, right and left ventricular function and the heart valves);
- radionuclide scan (MUGA scan) to measure left and/ or right ventricular ejection fraction;
- pulmonary function tests;
- exercise assessment to measure maximum oxygen uptake (VO_2max). This gives useful prognostic information and may be helpful in the timing of cardiac transplantation, particularly in young patients with dilated cardiomyopathy whose symptoms may not be particularly severe. It provides an objective assessment of the natural history of their disease. Once the VO_2max falls below 15 ml/kg/min, serious consideration needs

to be given to cardiac transplantation, even if symptoms are not particularly troublesome;[11]
- right heart catheterisation, to measure the TPG and/or the PVR. This is particularly important and may need to be repeated every 4–6 months, especially in patients whose levels are towards the upper end of the acceptable range;
- left heart catheterisation. It is important to exclude conventional cardiac surgery as a treatment option.

In some patients, other investigations may be required to address specific clinical questions – for example, PET scanning to assess the possibility of hibernating myocardium in patients with underlying coronary artery disease.

Mechanical circulatory support

Many patients die on the waiting list for cardiac transplantation, before a donor organ becomes available, because of the natural history of advanced myocardial disease. This may occur suddenly from a malignant ventricular arrhythmia.[11] If they are recognised to be at high risk of sudden cardiac death, these patients may be given additional time whilst awaiting a donor heart by the use of an implantable cardioverter-defibrillator. Alternatively, patients awaiting transplantation may die from progressive "pump" failure. Such patients, who experience a worsening of symptoms, may require hospital admission for the administration of intravenous inotropes. Although they will then have an increased priority category, many continue to decline and die before a donor organ becomes available. Consideration therefore has to be given to mechanical circulatory support to gain further time whilst awaiting a suitable donor.

The simplest form of mechanical circulatory support is the intraaortic balloon pump. This provides mechanical afterload reduction and produces augmentation of the cardiac function. The balloon pump can be inserted percutaneously and patients on such support usually qualify for transplantation in the highest urgency category. It does, however, have certain limitations and disadvantages: the patient must remain bedbound (with limited mobility and its attendant risks) and the amount of circulatory support provided is relatively limited. If an extended period of support is required (more than one week), there is an increased risk of related morbidity. Frequently, patients still die before an organ becomes available because of worsening cardiac decompensation. In view of these limitations, other techniques for mechanical circulatory support have been utilised and developed further. These include the use of ventricular assist devices, either of the left ventricle or of both ventricles, and the temporary use of the total artificial heart as a "bridge" to subsequent cardiac transplantation.

Extracorporeal pumps of various types can be used to provide substantial support of the circulation and can carry the whole systemic output. When the left ventricular output is supported, in many cases right ventricular failure develops. Therefore, in many instances, when ventricular assist is instituted it must be done in a biventricular configuration. Although the earlier assist systems required the patient to remain virtually bedbound, more recent developments in design have allowed an increasing degree of mobility. This has included a decrease in size of the assist devices and more sophisticated control systems. With such systems, however, there remains the ongoing risk of systemic infection and thromboembolic complications.

More recently, ventricular assist devices which are almost completely implantable have been developed. These include the Novacor and TCI

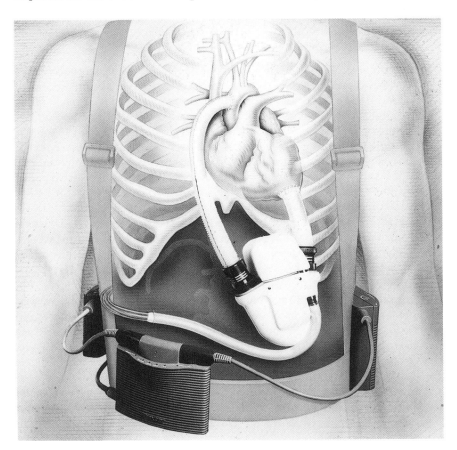

Fig 1.3 The Novacor implantable left ventricular assist device. There is an inlet conduit from the left ventricular cavity, and an outflow conduit back into the ascending aorta.

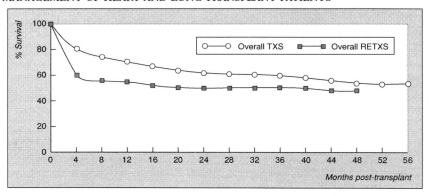

Fig 1.4 Actuarial survival curves for adult patients worldwide undergoing heart transplantation (overall TXS, all patients undergoing cardiac transplantation; overall RETXS, patients undergoing repeat cardiac transplantation).

systems (Figure 1.3). As well as allowing much greater patient mobility they can also provide support for much longer periods. The risks of infection and thromboembolism, however, remain an ongoing cause for concern.

The total artificial heart has also been used as a bridge to cardiac transplantation. The first successful case was reported in 1985.[12] As experience has increased with this class of device, it has become clear that there are significant risks involved. Mortality has occurred due to systemic infection and thromboembolic complications. When aggressive anti-coagulation regimes have been employed, morbidity and mortality from bleeding complications have been encountered.

As technical advances have been made in recent years with the various assist device systems, "bridging to transplantation" has become much more feasible in patients who develop worsening cardiac failure whilst awaiting cardiac transplantation. The results of cardiac transplantation have continued to improve in such patients and are now similar to those achieved in patients who do not require circulatory support preoperatively. The use of ventricular assist devices increases cardiac output and improves end-organ function, including renal and hepatic failure; this tends to reduce perioperative morbidity and mortality. Clearly, the use of ventricular assist devices as a "bridge" to transplantation is costly, and we need to be conscious of the cost-effectiveness of such an approach.

Patients who have undergone cardiac transplantation may eventually develop progressive deterioration in left ventricular function or widespread occlusive disease in the coronary circulation which is not amenable to revascularisation. In this situation, repeat cardiac transplantation may need to be considered. Generally, the results of repeat transplantation are not as good as those for the first operation (Figure 1.4). Once again, patients need to be thoroughly assessed; advanced renal dysfunction is often an issue in these circumstances. In certain carefully selected cases, repeat cardiac transplantation can be performed with encouraging results. We often face a conflict between the needs of an individual patient and the overall best use of available organs.

There is no doubt that cardiac transplantation is a highly effective treatment for many patients with endstage cardiac failure. The gap between the demand for transplantation and the supply of donor organs is likely to increase. We must make the best use of the organs available and aim to have as many donor organs as possible functioning five or 10 years after transplantation.

References

1 Evans RW, Manninen DL, Garrison LP et al. Donor availability as the primary determinant of the future of heart transplantation. *JAMA* 1986;**255**:1892.
2 International Society for Heart Transplantation Registry. Dallas, Texas, April 1990.
3 Consensus Trial Study Group. Effects of enalapril on mortality in severe congestive heart failure: results of the Co-operative North Scandinavian Enalapril Survival Study (CONSENSUS). *N Engl J Med* 1987;**316**:1429–35.
4 Buxton M, Acheson RM, Caine N, Gibson S, O'Brien B. *Costs and benefits of the heart transplant programmes at Harefield and Papworth Hospitals.* London: HMSO, 1985.
5 Carrier M, Emery RW, Riley JE et al. Cardiac transplantation in patients over 50 years of age. *J Am Coll Cardiol* 1986;**8**:285.
6 Dec GW, Semigran MJ, and Vlahakes GJ. Cardiac transplantation: current indications and limitations. *Transplant Proc* 1991;**23**:2095–106.
7 Rhenman MJ, Rhenman B, Icenogle T et al. Diabetes and heart transplantation. *J Heart Transplant* 1988;**7**:356.
8 Kirklin JK, Naftel DC, Kirklin JW et al. Pulmonary vascular resistance and the risk of heart transplantation. *J Heart Transplant* 1988;**7**:331.
9 Erickson KW, Costanzo-Nordin MR, O'Sullivan J et al. Influence of preoperative transpulmonary gradient on late mortality after orthotopic heart transplantation. *J Heart Transplant* 1990;**9**:526.
10 Edwards BS, Hunt SA, Fowler MB et al. Cardiac transplantion in patients with preexisting neoplastic diseases. *Am J Cardiol* 1990;**65**:501.
11 Stevenson LW. Selection and management of patients for cardiac transplantation. *Curr Opin Cardiol* 1994;**9**:315–25.
12 Copeland JG, Levinson MM, Smith R et al. The total artificial heart as a bridge to transplantation. A report of two cases. *JAMA* 1986;**256**:2991.

2 Selection of patients' suitability for lung transplant assessment

Paul A Corris

Introduction

The spectrum of lung transplantation procedures has evolved from heart-lung transplantation, which was first successfully performed at Stanford University in 1980, and it now additionally comprises lobar, single lung transplant and bilateral sequential single lung transplant procedures. More than 6500 lung transplantations have now been performed worldwide,[1] but the number of donor organs available for transplantation is far smaller than the number of patients with advanced lung or pulmonary vascular disease who may benefit. In order to optimise the best use of a rare resource and to ensure best outcome, it follows that certain criteria need to be applied carefully for the selection of candidates for lung transplantation. Doctors performing lung transplantations worldwide have recognised the need for a common approach and have recently agreed on broad guidelines to select suitable candidates for the procedure. The aim is to assist doctors treating patients with lung disease in identifying such candidates. Guidelines represent a general statement, and there will be room for individual centres to apply more specific guidelines for individual patients in specific circumstances. This chapter will focus on general health guidelines that all candidates for lung transplantation should meet and then on disease specific criteria that represent poor prognostic indicators, justifying consideration for transplantation.

General points regarding candidate selection

Lung transplantation is appropriate for patients who have declining lung function despite optimal medical treatment. Patients become candidates when no further medical or conventional surgery is available and survival is limited. Previously fit patients who become critically ill with acute illnesses are rarely candidates, and transplantation is much more suited to patients with chronic respiratory disease. It should be recognised that up to 40% of patients may die while on an active waiting list for transplantation and the median time spent on a waiting list before transplantation varies from one to two years, depending upon centre and indication.[2] The registry of the International Society for Heart and Lung Transplantation now has data that show that older patients have a significantly worse outcome than younger patients,[1] and accordingly the following age limits are suggested (Box 2.1).

Heart lung transplantation: age ≤55 years
Sequential single lung transplantation: age ≤60 years
Single lung transplantation: age ≤65 years

The age limits given above are a pragmatic approach to achieving a balance, but it is recognised that individual consideration should be given in appropriate cases.

General medical considerations

Function of other vital organs

Renal disease

Lung transplantation imposes a major stress on a patient and will be successful only if all other major organs are functioning well. Currently, two of the major drugs used as the basis for immunosuppression — cyclosporin

---

Box 2.1 *Contraindications to lung transplantation*

- Weight outside range >70%, <130% Ideal Body Weight (IBW)
- Bilateral pleurodesis for cardiopulmonary bypass candidates
- Age
    >65 for single lung transplantation
    >60 for bilateral single lung transplantation
    >55 for heart and lung transplantation
- Psychosocial stability
- Tobacco use within six months
- Intrinsic renal disease
- Significant peripheral vascular disease
- Impaired left heart function unless considered for heart and lung transplantation
- Symptomatic osteoporosis
- Severe chest wall deformity
- Sputum with panresistant bacteria or aspergilloma
- Hepatitis B or C infection and liver damage
- Malignancy precluding long term survival
- HIV +ve

---

and tacrolimus are nephrotoxic,[3] and, accordingly, candidates require good renal function. Experience has shown that renal failure is accelerated in patients with pre-existing abnormal renal function before the introduction of nephrotoxic immunosuppression.[4] As a consequence, serum creatinine concentrations in all candidates should be in the normal range, and patients should have a creatinine clearance of 50 ml/min or greater.

Hepatic disease

Azathioprine is hepatotoxic, and hepatic function should be preserved, particularly with regard to synthetic function as assessed by serum albumin and normal prothrombin time. Some diseases, such as cystic fibrosis and $\alpha 1$ anti-trypsin deficiency, are associated with coexistent hepatic disease and elevations in enzymes such as alkaline phosphatase. Provided that synthetic function is preserved and that there is no portal hypertension, patients may remain candidates for lung transplantation alone. A small number of patients with significant intrinsic hepatic disease may be considered for combined liver and lung transplantation. A raised bilirubin concentration in patients with primary pulmonary hypertension requires careful investigation since it may represent hepatic cirrhosis as a result of chronic right heart failure.[5]

Cardiac disease

Candidates should be free of coronary artery disease of prognostic significance because of the risk of perioperative myocardial infarction.[6] A few patients have undergone preoperative angioplasty or perioperative coronary artery bypass grafting at the same time as lung transplantation. A patient with significant left ventricular systolic or diastolic dysfunction is not a candidate for lung transplantation alone, but may be a candidate for heart and lung transplantation. Many candidates for lung transplantation will have pulmonary hypertension as a result of chronic hypoxic remodelling of their pulmonary vasculature and as a consequence have a dilated right ventricle with abnormal function. Studies have shown improvements in right sided haemodynamics after single lung transplantation, with normalisation of right ventricular volumes.[7] Successful single lung transplantation has been carried out in a patient with a right ventricular ejection fraction of only 12%, although mean ejection fractions for a series of patients undergoing single lung transplantation or sequential single lung transplantation were 31% and 38% respectively.[8] The right ventricle has great capacity to show improved function after lung transplant surgery, and the presence of cor pulmonale is not a contraindication for either single lung transplantation or sequential single lung transplantation.

Despite the current best efforts to detect cardiac disease before transplant surgery, heart failure has been responsible for 9% of all deaths in the first 90 days after lung transplantation.[9] It is the third leading cause of death after infection (32%) and primary allograft failure (12%). Thus, severe cardiac disease is a relative contraindication to isolated lung transplantation, but each situation should be assessed individually. Heart and lung transplantation may be considered when significant cardiac disease is present.

Nutritional state

Many patients reaching the end stage for chronic pulmonary disease show symptoms of cachexia and malnutrition.[10] Nutritional status has emerged as a prognostic indicator in thoracic transplantation, and candidates should be 70%–130% of their ideal body weight. All recipients lose weight in the first week after transplantation and severe nutritional deficiency before the operation weakens the ability to withstand the rigors of the postoperative period and increases patients' susceptibility to infection and poor wound healing. Obesity, however, increases surgical risk, predisposing to atelectasis and impairing postoperative mobility that is essential after lung transplantation. The recipients of early unsuccessful transplants were all bed bound, and most transplant centres now require that recipients are capable of self care and of participating in exercise rehabilitation to help maintain muscle bulk and physical fitness. The ability to mobilise quickly after surgery is a key factor in postoperative recovery.

Infection

Potential candidates with active extrapulmonary sepsis should have the infection irradicated before they are accepted for transplantation. The one area of debate relates to sinusitis in patients with cystic fibrosis. Some lung transplant programmes require sinus surgery, followed by irrigation with tobramycin, in an attempt to lower the colonising load of infection.[11] Other programmes have no requirements. No prospective study comparing outcomes has been carried out to substantiate the benefit of sinus surgery.

Aspergillus in the sputum of a prospective candidate is regarded by some as a relative contraindication, but treatment with itraconazole or nebulised amphotericin can reduce colonisation in most cases. The presence of a subpleural aspergilloma, on the other hand, does mitigate against successful transplantation because of the risk of contaminating the pleural space with aspergillus during surgery.

Infection with HIV, hepatitis B when virus DNA positive, and hepatitis C with histological evidence of liver damage[12] renders a potential candidate as unsuitable. High dose steroid treatment leads to increase in hepatitis C viraemia in patients following transplantation[12] with recurrence of hepatitis.[12,13]

Previous colonisation by atypical mycobacteria is not an absolute contraindication for transplantation, and cases should be considered on an individual basis. Special care should be given when a single lung transplant is considered. Adequately treated *Mycobacterium tuberculosis* is not a contraindication.

Malignancy

No patient should be considered a candidate for transplantation with evidence of malignancy in the previous two years, with the exception of basal cell or squamous cell carcinoma of the skin. Recent data on recurrence of tumour after transplantation suggest that a waiting period of at least five years is prudent for solid organ tumours.[14]

Osteoporosis

Symptomatic osteoporosis is emerging as an important contraindication to successful transplantation, and the potential risk to long term outcome should be assessed on a case by case basis.[15]

Musculoskeletal pain after lung transplantation impairs the rehabilitation of recipients, which increases the risks of secondary complications such as atelectasis and pneumonia. Bone mineral density should be measured in all potential recipients, given the increased risk of osteoporosis in patients with chronic respiratory disease and treatment with bisphosphonates instituted in patients whose bone mineral density falls below two standard deviations of the age and sex related mean.

Systemic disease

Patients with diabetes or connective tissue disease may be accepted for transplantation, providing the underlying problem is well controlled and significant end organ damage of other organs has not occurred. The literature provides limited guidance, but it seems that the outcome of patients with connective tissue disease does not differ from that of patients with pure respiratory disease.[16]

Peripheral vascular disease is a relative contraindication to lung transplantation. Ischaemic symptoms from lower extremity vascular disease can preclude an acceptable level of rehabilitation, and the haemodynamic instability may lead to substantial risk of occlusion of a blood vessel. Systemic hypertension and peptic ulcer disease should be optimally controlled before assessment.

Steroid therapy

Patients may be considered suitable candidates for transplantation even though they are treated with oral corticosteroids. The literature suggests that there are no greater risks, provided that there is no evidence of severe corticosteroid induced myopathy, osteoporosis, or skin thinning, and the daily dose is 20 mg or less.[17]

Mechanical ventilation

Although lung transplantation has been performed in people who were on mechanical ventilation, there is a 30 fold increased risk of a poor outcome for people requiring intubation before transplantation.[18] The use of nocturnal support by nasal bi-level positive airway pressure does not carry a similar risk and can be considered as a bridge to transplantation in unstable patients.[19] Patients or candidates should generally not receive mechanical ventilation when the need for this intervention is solely a result of the progression of the underlying disease.

Pleura

There is a risk of haemorrhage when native lungs are removed in the presence of pleural scars or adhesions. Clearly there is a gradation of risk from scarring due to previous open lung biopsy by limited thoracotomy and previous total pleurectomy. The latter remains a contraindication to heart and lung transplantation because of the systemic anticoagulation required for cardiopulmonary bypass.

A prior thoracotomy that results in a significant reduction in the size of the hemithorax may preclude the use of that hemithorax for a lung transplant. The exception is reduction pneumoplasty in patients with emphysema, where successful lung transplantation has been carried out after such surgery.[20] Open lung biopsy and an uncomplicated lobectomy do not generally reduce the hemithorax significantly and are not contra-indications to successful transplant surgery.

Psychosocial stability

Psychological and social stability of the candidate and family and his/her carers is important.[21] The time before and even after the transplantation is filled with new and potentially debilitating stresses. Before surgery, candidates are concerned about living long enough to receive a transplant and the emotional burden of their illness on their carers. After surgery recipients are concerned about living as long as possible by avoiding complications, such as infection and rejection. The post-transplant medical regimen is rigorous, with a need to monitor the allograft carefully, to take medication that has side effects, and repeatedly to undergo procedures that may be unpleasant, such as fibreoptic bronchoscopy. In the United States financial concerns remain important. The cost of medication and health-care coverage can cause significant anxiety and worry. The availability of health insurance can restrict occupational, residential, and lifestyle choices. In order to maintain health insurance, some recipients cannot return to gainful employment, and others cannot change jobs. All of this takes a toll on candidates, recipients, and their carers.

Examples of psychosocial instability include: the absence of a strong family structure; a history of non-compliance; and misuse of alcohol or drugs, such as narcotics or tranquillisers. As stress can precipitate psychiatric illness, a history of a major psychiatric illness or the occurrence of one during the waiting period – such as depression, suicide attempt, chronic anxiety or other neurosis – is a relative contraindication to transplantation. The risk is increased that the recipient may not be able to take care of the allograft after transplantation. Thus, the psychosocial situation of prospective candidates is carefully assessed during the evaluation and reassessed repeatedly while waiting for a donor to become available.

Tobacco abuse

Tobacco use after-transplantation makes an assessment of the allograft more difficult. In non-smokers, long term allograft dysfunction can only be the result of infection, rejection, or complications at the airway anastomosis. In cigarette smokers, dysfunction can also be the result of bronchospasm, airway irritation, infectious bronchitis, and respiratory bronchiolitis, or both. In recipients of single lung transplants, these effects can occur in the allograft and in the native lung.

Patients must abstain from cigarette smoking for six months before being accepted as a candidate for a lung transplant. Compliance with smoking cessation in the pre-evaluation and waiting period can be monitored by random testing of the urine and saliva or both for cotinine, which is a breakdown product of nicotine.[22] While enough exposure to second hand smoke can cause cotinine to be present in the urine,[23] candidates for lung transplantation should not be in this type of environment. A positive result during the pre-evaluation period should result in postponement of assessment for lung transplantation.

Chest wall deformity

Chest wall deformity due to kyphosis and scoliosis or both may be a result of congenital spine defects, acquired for idiopathic reasons, or secondary to neuromuscular, intrathoracic, or vertebral disease, such as after thoracoplasty, pneumonectomy, or tuberculosis of the spine. Independent of aetiology and type of underlying pulmonary disease, these deformities can adversely affect the ventilatory capacity of the lung both before and after transplant surgery.[22,23] This effectively restricts the rehabilitation potential of affected candidates and especially recipients, particularly during the crucial early days after transplant surgery. Because the effect of chest wall deformity on the ventilatory function of the lung is variable and can be difficult to assess when cardiopulmonary disease is present, each case must be evaluated individually. A chest wall deformity should be a contraindication to lung transplantation if there is a substantial risk that it will result in ventilatory failure after transplant surgery.

Disease specific guidelines

Background

In addition to the general guidelines just mentioned, there are some disease specific guidelines that can help to identify opportunity for a candidate for lung transplant surgery. The information for these disease specific considerations comes from published observations regarding the natural history of different types of lung diseases, the factors that influence this natural history, the clinical characteristics of candidates who survive long enough to receive an allograft compared with those who die while waiting, and the anticipated survival following lung transplantation. After lung transplantation, recipient survival has been reported to be 67–72% at one year, 57–64% at two years and 49–57% at three years after transplant surgery. After heart and lung transplantation, recipient survival has been reported to be 56–61% at one year, 45–53% at two years and 40–49% at three years after transplantation. In the registry of the International Society for Heart and Lung Transplantation significantly fewer recipients of single, but not bilateral lung transplants, who had underlying pulmonary hypertension or fibrosis survived, compared with recipients who had underlying emphysema.[1] In the St Louis international registry, survival was lower for recipients who had underlying pulmonary hypertension and pulmonary fibrosis, compared with those who had emphysema. Thus in all registries there is a trend for recipients with emphysema to fare best while recipients with pulmonary hypertension or fibrosis do less well after lung transplantation (Box 2.2).

Box 2.2 *Selection guidelines for lung transplantation*

General indications
Advanced pulmonary parenchymal and/or vascular disease with:
    Projected life expectancy <2 years
    NYHA III and IV functional level with rehabilitation potential
Disease specific indications
    Idiopathic pulmonary fibrosis
        VC (Vital Capacity) <65% of predicted
        Patient does not respond to treatment with steroids
    Cystic fibrosis
        FEV_1 (Forced Expiratory Volume in one second) <30% of predicted
        and or PaO_2 at rest <7.3 kPa
    Primary pulmonary hypertension
        Symptomatic disease
        Failed response to continuous intravenous epoprostenol
    Emphysema
        Post-bronchodilator FEV_1 <25% of predicted

Retransplantation

These candidates are lung recipients whose allograft is failing. Early in the period post transplant surgery, this is usually a result of non-function of the allograft, which is often caused by an ischaemic reperfusion lung injury that results in diffuse alveolar damage – the histologic equivalent of the adult respiratory distress syndrome.[23] Late after transplantation, the usual cause of allograft failure is obliterative bronchiolitis (OB), which is a histologic manifestation of chronic allograft rejection.[24] The success of retransplantation compared with first time transplantation is poor, particularly when performed for allografts that fail in the first two weeks after transplantation.[8] For allografts that fail more than two weeks after transplantation, the one year survival for heart and lung allografts is 28% and for lung allografts is 39%. Recipients with failing allografts due to OB can be listed for retransplantation, but they should only undergo lung transplantation and should not receive added advantage over other candidates with other types of end stage lung disease.

Idiopathic pulmonary fibrosis

The mean survival rate for patients with idiopathic pulmonary fibrosis at two years after diagnosis has been reported to be 80%.[26] When subsets of patients were examined, the two year survival rate after diagnosis was lower for men (60%) compared with women (80%), lower with increasing age (60% for 60–69 years v 75% for <50 years), lower with increasing radiographic infiltrates, and lower with more histologic fibrosis.[27] More importantly, the two year survival rate in patients who did not respond to 20–40 mg of prednisolone/day in 2–8 weeks with a >10% increase in the vital capacity was only 33% for patients with dyspnoea for activities of daily living, only 20% for patients with initial vital capacity <60% of predicted, and only 10% for patients with an initial artery pressure of oxygen (PaO_2) on room air of (<60 mm Hg).[28] In another study, the two year survival was only 50% in patients with an initial vital capacity (VC) <67% of predicted who did not respond to treatment with immunosuppressive medication within 4–6 weeks with an increase >10% in the vital capacity that was maintained for at least one year.[29] Patients with idiopathic pulmonary fibrosis should be referred for lung transplantation when the vital capacity approaches 65% of predicted and there has been no response to immunosuppressive treatment.

Candidates with idiopathic pulmonary fibrosis are more likely to die waiting, compared with candidates with cystic fibrosis or primary pulmonary hypertension (PPH) and, especially, candidates with emphysema. This is most probably because these patients are referred late in the course of their illness, when the disease is advanced. Patients should be considered candidates for transplant if they meet the ventilatory criteria even though they may not yet be markedly hypercapnic or hypoxaemic.

Transplant centres are happy to evaluate patients with idiopathic pulmonary fibrosis early in the course of their disease, and doctors should not hesitate to refer otherwise suitable patients if there is failure to maintain lung function despite systemic treatment with corticosteroids, including exercise oxygen desaturation, even if vital capacity is greater than 65% of predicted.

Coexistent pulmonary conditions for which the patient should be evaluated before referral are bronchial carcinoma and coexistent bronchiectatic areas colonised by bacteria. A high resolution computerised tomography scan is useful in assessing these issues. Treatment should be optimised, and this should include the withdrawal of steroids where no benefit has been achieved.

Systemic disease with pulmonary fibrosis

Pulmonary fibrosis is a common lung pathology in a number of systemic diseases – for example, scleroderma, rheumatoid arthritis, sarcoidosis, post-chemotherapy. In patients with these diagnoses, the manifestations of the underlying process are highly variable, and each patient should be considered on an individual basis. In general, evidence of quiescent systemic disease is required. It is necessary for all patients to meet general selection criteria and to have failed optimum medical therapy to be considered for lung transplantation. The criteria for timing of selection for transplant listed above should be followed.

Cystic fibrosis

For patients with cystic fibrosis, the risk of death within two years has been reported to be about 50% when the vital capacity falls to <40% of predicted, the forced expiratory volume to <30% of predicted, the room air PaO_2 is <55 mm Hg (7.3 kPa), the $PaCO_2$ is > 50 mm Hg (6.6 kPa) and the height:weight ratio is <70%.[30] Within these considerations, the risk of death is greater for women less than 18 years of age.[31] The two year survival after lung transplantation for cystic fibrosis exceeds that value, and patients with cystic fibrosis should therefore be referred when they reach this profile. Patients should be considered candidates for transplantation if they meet the spirometric criteria, even though they may not yet be hypercapnic or hypoxic. Other guidelines for referral include an increased frequency of hospitalisation, an unexpected rapid fall in FEV_1, massive haemoptysis uncontrolled by bronchial embolisation, and increasing cachexia despite optimal medical management.

Patients with cystic fibrosis have special problems related to the microbiology of their pulmonary secretions, particularly with respect to resistant organisms.[32] Controversy exists as to the outcome of patients colonised with multiply resistant *Pseudomonas aeruginosa* and *Burkholderia cepacia* (biologically, *B cepacia* is inherently multiply resistant). The following definitions may be used to categorise the resistance of pseudomonal and related organisms.[33]

- A multiply resistant organism is resistant to all agents in two of the following classes of antibiotics: the β-lactams, aminoglycosides and/or quinolones.
- A panresistant organism is resistant in vitro to all groups of antibiotics.

A substantial number of patients will have organisms that are panresistant in vitro. However, in vitro resistance does not equate with in vivo resistance. Different combinations of antibiotics may function synergistically in vivo. Thus multiple resistance is not a contraindication to transplantation in this group of patients. Colonisation with panresistant organisms should be considered a relative contraindication to transplantation because of concern about long term outcomes in these patients. Occasionally specialised testing of different combinations of antibiotics against organisms considered to be panresistant to the usual antibiotic regimens may demonstrate sensitivity to new drug combinations (synergy testing). Patients with presumed panresistant organisms should be referred to a transplant centre capable of antibiotic sensitivity testing, and each patient should be assessed on an individual basis. Listing of such patients should be determined on the basis of individual centre experience.

Microbiologic review of the sputum listed patients should be done on a periodic basis, for example, every three months, or if intercurrent antibiotic treatment has been necessary.

Pulmonary hypertension without congenital heart disease

Severe pulmonary hypertension occurs as a primary process or as a secondary manifestation of another disease. Typical causes of secondary pulmonary hypertension include thromboembolic disease, venoocclusive disease, capillary haemagiomatosis, medication related, and collagen vascular disease. Patients with these diagnoses generally have a poor prognosis.[34]

Advances in long term vasodilator treatment, using continuous intravenous epoprostenol have recently shown encouraging results in patients with primary pulmonary hypertension.[35] Less information is available in patients with pulmonary hypertension as a secondary manifestation of other disease; but studies in selected patients are ongoing. In selected cases surgical therapy – including atrial septostomy in PPH or thromboendartectomy in chronic thromboembolic disease – have been reported to improve symptoms and survival.[36,37]

24

Potential candidates for lung transplant with a diagnosis of primary pulmonary hypertension should be evaluated by a centre with experience in vasodilator therapy, and all patients should be evaluated for vasodilator therapy and other medical or surgical interventions before they are considered for transplant surgery. The following criteria should be met to consider a patient within the transplant window.

- Symptomatic, progressive disease which despite optimal medical and surgical treatment or both, leaves the patient in New York Heart Association functional class III or IV (NYHA III or IV). Where available, prostacyclin should be considered the gold standard for medical vasodilator therapy if there is no objective indication that calcium channel blockers may be useful.
- Useful haemodynamic indices in assessing the failure of optimal medical treatment include a cardiac index of less than 2 l/min/m² a right atrial pressure of more than 15 mm Hg, a mean pulmonary artery pressure greater than 85 mm Hg, and a mixed venous oxygen saturation of less than 63%.

Advanced liver disease can be associated with pulmonary hypertension.[38] In a limited number of centres with multiorgan transplant expertise, selected patients with liver and lung disease may be candidates for liver and lung transplants.[39] In each case, the candidate should meet all the criteria for selection for the individual transplant.

Pulmonary hypertension secondary to congenital heart disease (Eisenmenger's syndrome)

Pulmonary hypertension in patients with congenital heart disease manifests itself differently prognostically than in patients with other types of pulmonary hypertension.

Haemodynamically, similar pulmonary artery pressures are associated with better cardiac function and lower right atrial pressures and a better prognosis. Predictors of survival are less reliable. The role of vasodilator therapy in pretransplant management of these patients is not yet clear.

Patients may be considered for transplant assessment when they have severe, progressive symptoms with function at NYHA III or NYHA IV despite optimal medical management.

In conclusion, this chapter has attempted to cover the main indications and selection criteria for potential candidates for lung transplantation. The criteria represent a pragmatic approach to the literature concerning both prognosis in patients with pulmonary disease and outcome following lung transplantation. The guidelines should be regarded as guidelines, and there is always room for discussion regarding the merits of an individual patient with the transplanting surgeon/doctor.

References

1 Hosenpud JD, Bennett LE, Keck BM, Fiol B, Novick RJ. The Registry of the International Society for Heart and Lung Transplantation: fourteenth official report – 1997. *J Heart Lung Transplant* 1997;**16**:691–712.
2 *1996 annual report of the US scientific registry for transplant recipients and the organ procurement and transplantation network – transplant data 1988–1995.* UNOS, Richmond VA, and the Division of Transplantation, Bureau of Health Resources Development, Health Resources and Services Administration, US Dept of Health and Human Services, Rockville, MD.
3 Zaltzman JS, Pei Y, Maurer J, Patterson A, Cattran DC. Cyclosporine nephrotoxicity in lung transplant recipients. *Transplantation* 1992;**54**:875–8.
4 Myers BD, Ross J, Newton LN, Luetscher J, Perlroth M. Cyclosporine-associated chronic nephropathy. *N Engl J Med* 1984;**311**:699–705.
5 Kramer MR, Marshall SE, Tiroke A, Lewiston NJ, Starnes VA, Theodore J. Clinical significance of hyperbilirubinemia in patients with pulmonary hypertension undergoing heart-lung transplantation. *J Heart Lung Transplant* 1991;**10**:317–321.
6 Thaik CM, Semigran JM, Ginns L, Wain JC, Dec GW. Evaluation of ischaemic heart disease in potential lung transplant recipient. *J Heart Lung Transplant* 1995;**14**:257–266.
7 Doig C, Corris PA, Hilton CJ, Dark JH, Bexton RS. The effect of single lung transplantation on pulmonary hypertension in patients with end stage fibrosing lung disease. *British Heart Journal* 1991;**66**:431–434.
8 Morrison DL, Maurer JR and Grossman RF. Preoperative assessment for lung transplantation. *Clinics Chest Med* 1990;**2**:207–215.
9 Pohl M, Cooper J. The international status of lung transplantation. *Am J Respir Crit Care Med* 1996;**153**:A829.
10 Hunter AMB, Carey MA and Larsh HW. The nutritional status of patients with chronic obstructive pulmonary disease. *Am Rev Respir Dis* 1981;**124**:376–381.
11 Davidson TM, Murphy C, Mitchell M, Smith C, Light M. Management of chronic sinusitis in cystic fibrosis. *Laryngoscope* 1995;**105**:354–358.
12 Starzl TE, Demetris AJ, Van Thiel DH. Liver transplantation. *N Engl J Med* 1989;**321**:1014–1022.
13 Periera BJG, Wright TL, Schmid CH, Levy AS. The impact of pretransplantation hepatitis C infection on the outcome of renal transplantation. *Transplantation* 1995;**60**:799–805.
14 Penn I. Incidence and treatment of neoplasia after transplantation. *J Heart Lung Transplant* 1993;**12**:S328–S336.
15 Aris RM, Neuringer IP, Weiner MA, Egan TM, Ontjes D. Severe osteoporosis before and after lung transplantation. *Chest* 1996;**109**:1176–83.
16 Levine SM, Anzueto AR, Peters JI, Calhoon JH, Jenkinson SG, Bryan CL. Single lung transplantation in patients with systemic disease. *Chest* 1994;**105**:837–841.
17 Novick RJ, Meukis AH, McKenzie N, Reid KR, Pflugfelder PW, Kostuk WJ, Ahmad D. The safety of low-dose prednisolone before and immediately after heart-lung transplantation. *Ann Thorac Surg* 1991;**51**:642–645.
18 Hosenpud JD, Novick RJ, Bennett LE, Keck BM, Fiol B, Daily OP. The Registry of the International Society for Heart and Lung Transplantation: thirteenth official report. *J Heart Lung Transplant* 1996;**15**:655–674.
19 Hodson ME, Madden BP, Steven MH, Tsang VT, Yacoub MH. Noninvasive mechanical ventilation for cystic fibrosis patients – a potential bridge to transplantation. *Eur Respir J* 1991;**4**:524–527.
20 Zenati M, Keenan RJ, Landreneau RJ, Paradis IL, Ferson PF, Griffith BP. Lung reduction as bridge to lung transplantation in pulmonary emphysema., *Ann Thorac Surg* 1995;**59**:1581–1583.
21 Olbrisch ME, Levenson JL. Psychosocial assessment of organ transplant candidates. *Psychosomatics* 1995;**36**:226–243.
22 Benowitz NL. Pharmacologic aspects of cigarette smoking and nicotine addiction. *N Engl J Med* 1988;**319**:1075–1078.
23 Matsukura S, Taminato T, Kitano N, Seino Y, Hamada H, Uchihashi M, Nakajima H, Hirata Y. Effects of environmental tobacco smoke on urinary cotinine excretion in non-smokers. Evidence for passive smoking. *N Engl J Med* 1984;**311**:828–832.

24 Kerem E, Reisman J, Corey M, Canny GJ, Levison H. Prediction of mortality in patients with cystic fibrosis. *N Engl J Med* 1992;**326**:1187–1191.
25 Sharples L, Hathaway T, Dennis C, Caine N, Higenbottam T, Wallwork J. Prognosis of patients with cystic fibrosis awaiting heart and lung transplantation. *J Heart Lung Transplant* 1993;**12**:669–674.
26 Carrington CB, Gaensler EA, Coutu RE, Fitzgerald MX, Gupta RT. Natural history and treated course of usual and desquamative interstitial pneumonia. *N Engl J Med* 1978;**298**:801–809.
27 Turner-Warwick M, Burrows B, Johnson A. Cryptogenic fibrosing alveolitis: Clinical features and their influence on survival. *Thorax* 1972;**27**:535–542.
28 Stack BHR, Choo-Kang YFJ, Heard BE. The prognosis of cryptogenic fibrosing alveolitis. *Thorax* 1972;**27**:535–542.
29 Rudd RM, Haslam PL, Turner-Warwick M. Cryptogenic fibrosing alveolitis: Relationships of pulmonary physiology and bronchoalveolar lavage to response to treatment and prognosis. *Am Rev Respir Dis* 1981;**124**:1–8.
30 Kerem E, Reisman J, Corey M, Canny GJ, Levison H. Prediction of mortality in patients with cystic fibrosis. *N Eng J Med* 1992;**326**:1187–91.
31 Dodge JA, Morison S, Lewis PA, Colest EC, Geddes D, Russell G *et al*. Cystic fibrosis in the United Kingdom 1968–1988: incidence population and survival. *Paediatric Perinat Epidem* 1993;7:157–66.
32 Aris RM, Gilligan PH, Neuringer IP, Gott KK, Rea J, Yankaskas JR. The effects of panresistant bacteria in cystic fibrosis patients on lung transplant outcome. *Am J Res Crit Care Med* 1997;**155**:1699–704.
33 *Microbiology and Infectious Diseases in Cystic Fibrosis*. From North American Cystic Fibrosis Foundation Concepts in Care Consensus Conference 1994;5:1–25.
34 D'Alonzo GE, Barst RJ, Ayers SM, Bergofsky EH, Brundage BH, Detre KM *et al*. Survival in patients with primary pulmonary hypertension. *Ann Intern Med* 1991;**115**:343–349.
35 Barst RJ, Rubin LJ, Long WA, McGoon MD, Rich S, Badesch DB *et al*. A comparison of continuous intravenous epoprostenol (prostacyclin) with conventional therapy for primary pulmonary hypertension. *N Engl J Med* 1996;**334**:296–301.
36 Kerstein D, Levy PS, Hsu DT, Hurdof AJ, Gersony WM, Barst RJ. Blade balloon atrial septostomy in patients with severe primary pulmonary hypertension. *Circulation* 1995;**91**:2028–35.
37 Fedullo PF, Auger WR, Channick RN, Moser KM, Jamieson SW. Chronic thromboembolic pulmonary hypertension. *Clin Chest Med* 1995;**16**:353–74.
38 Mandell MS, Groves BM. Pulmonary hypertension in chronic liver disease. *Clin Chest Med* 1996;**16**:17–33.
39 Wallwork J, Calne RY, Williams R. Transplantation of liver, heart and lungs for primary biliary cirrhosis and primary pulmonary hypertension. *Lancet* 1987;2:182.
40 Cooper JD, Patterson GA, Sundaresan RS, Trulock EP, Yusen RD, Pohl MS *et al*. Results of 150 consecutive bilateral lung volume reduction procedures in patients with severe emphysema. *J Thorac Cardiovasc Surg* 1996;**112**:1319–30.
41 Anthonisen NR. Prognosis in chronic obstructive pulmonary disease: results from multicentre clinical trials. *Am Rev Resp Dis* 1989;**140**:S95–9.
42 Gray-Donald K, Gibbons L, Shapiro SH, Macklem PT, Martin JG. Nutritional status and mortality in chronic obstructive pulmonary disease. *Am J Respir Crit Care Med* 1996;**153**:961–6.
43 Seersholm N, Dirksen A, Kok-Jensen A. Airways obstruction and two year survival in patients with severe alpha 1-antitrypsin deficiency. *Eur Resp J* 1994;7:1985–7.
44 Bando K, Paradis IL, Keenan RJ, Yousem SA, Komatsu K, Konishi Hr *et al*. Comparison of outcomes afte single and bilateral lung transplantation for obstructive lung disease. *J Heart Lung Transplant* 1995;**14**:692–8.
45 Smith CM. Patient selection, evaluation and preoperative management for lung transplant candidates. *Clin Chest Med* 1997;**18**:183–97.
46 Connors Jr AF, Dawson NV, Thomas C, Harrell Jr FE, Desbiens N, Fulkerson WJ *et al*. Outcomes following acute exacerbation of severe chronic obstructive lung disease. *Am J Respir Crit Care Med* 1996;**154**:959–67.

3 Organ donation for heart and lung transplantation

A El Gamel, J J Egan

Introduction

Over the last 30 years, the field of organ transplantation has advanced from an experimental curiosity to an established treatment option for patients with irreversible organ failure. The demand for viable human organs for transplantation continues to exceed the supply. Prime quality organs are a scarce resource, best fostered by doctors and surgeons educated in the principles of donor management, and by the provision of expert organ retrieval teams. This chapter will explore current issues related to thoracic organ donation and the management of potential donors.

The national organisation of organ retrieval and placement

A novel zoning system for the allocation and retrieval of donor organs began in the United Kingdom on 1 November 1993. There are eight adult cardiac zones and one centre, Great Ormond Street (London), which specialises particularly in paediatric transplantation. In addition there are seven zones aligned to centres undertaking lung transplantation, including Harefield, Papworth, Manchester, Newcastle, Birmingham, St George's (London) and Sheffield. The aim of the zonal procurement was to benefit both the retrieval teams and the donating centre by:

(a) allowing shorter and predictable retrieval journeys
(b) promoting familiarity between retrieval teams and donor centres
(c) standardisation of retrieval practice.

This policy has largely achieved its goals over the United Kingdom in the past four years.[1]

Optimising the donor pool

Initiatives to reduce road traffic accidents and strategies for the management of systemic hypertension have reduced the number of

28

potential organ donors.[2] Other factors, including a lack of intensive care beds, promote an environment in which some potential donors, on the basis of prognostic criteria, may not be ventilated. Concurrently the demand for lung and heart transplantation has increased exponentially. Up to 30% of patients awaiting lung and heart transplantation die because of apparent shortages of donor organs.

A variety of strategies to increase the supply of organs for transplantation have been proposed:

(a) education programmes optimising staff communication skills in order to minimise refusal by relatives
(b) early identification of potential donors
(c) organ care initiatives to avoid non-procurement of suitable organs and to prevent deterioration of initially suitable organs.

In order to facilitate donation, education strategies aimed at nursing and medical staff potentially involved in the management of potential donors have been advocated. An education programme targeted at intensive care and accident and emergency staff has been undertaken under the auspices of the European Donor Hospital Education Programme.[3] This programme has demonstrated encouraging results, but further evaluation is required. In the United Kingdom, regional coordinators have enacted education strategies by establishing close links with nurses in individual intensive care units and completing teaching sessions aimed at intensive care, anaesthetic and theatre staff.

Donor action strategies have also been piloted with encouraging results.[3] This entails reviewing medical records from an intensive care unit in order to estimate the potential rate of donation in comparison to the actual rate of donation. Although staff may feel under scrutiny, such a review may highlight strengths and weaknesses in the donation process and may facilitate improved rates of donation.

The early identification of donors is another important strategy to increase donor rates. The aim of the strategy is to facilitate appropriate communication with the family and initiate skilled donor management at an early stage. In Spain an individual transplant coordinator is allocated to each hospital, and he or she is responsible for identifying potential donors.[4] This has resulted in a 40% increase in the rate of organ donation, increasing from 14.3 per million of the population in 1989 to 21.7 donors per million of the population in 1992. Early identification has resulted in improved organ retrieval rates increasing by 81% during the same period, and the rate of cardiac transplantation increased by 162%.

Similar strategies have been enacted in Pennsylvania, United States, where after a donor has been identified, specifically skilled people are sent to the hospital to facilitate donation.[5] There were also indirect incentives to both the hospital and the relatives to facilitate organ donation. This combined strategy has resulted in an overall increase in organ donation rates from 21 to 27 donors per million population. In Pennsylvania, financial incentives encompass help with funeral expenses and a punitive charge to the hospital if a donor was not referred. In the United Kingdom donor intensive care units receive £1000 for costs.[2] In contrast, intensive care units in Spain are reimbursed up to as much as £40 000.

Optimising donor management in order to maximise organ retrieval is another important aspect of improving the rate of transplantation. In a study of 150 potential multiorgan donations, 35% (n = 52) were unsuitable for heart donation when the basic acceptance criteria were applied.[6] Careful invasive monitoring and hormone therapy, however, resulted in over 80% of these "unsuitable" cardiac donors being subsequently transplanted. Eighty-four per cent of the recipients of these "unsuitable" heart donations were alive at a minimum of one year follow up.

Standards for lung donation may also be more flexible. A retrospective study has suggested that marginal lung donors not fulfilling standard criteria may be utilised with acceptable survival for the recipients.[7] Of 44 donors failing one of the standard criteria for donation there was no disadvantage in terms of survival (86%) compared with recipients of lung transplants fulfilling all the criteria (83%). This study does not, however, specifically redefine new criteria. The implication is that, after careful assessment by an experienced team, the strict application of standard criteria can be relaxed to include more marginal donors.

All the strategies outlined emphasise that highlighting transplantation and optimising donor management will potentially facilitate increased rates of both organ donation and utilisation. However, the best cost effective vehicle for increasing both organ donation and utilisation remains to be determined by the long term follow up of the initiatives described.

Brain stem death

History

Central to clinical transplantation is the acceptance of brain stem death, both legally and medically. The concept of brain stem death is relatively recent in origin. In 1959 French doctors showed, for the first time, massive brain autolysis in a patient maintained by mechanical ventilatory support.[8] Problems with the medicolegal definition of death prevented Hardy from using a human donor for heart transplantation in the early 1960s and set the stage for his use of a chimpanzee heart to replace a human heart in 1964. Barnard's report of the first human to human heart transplant in 1967 describes graft removal after five minutes of cardiac asystole and apnoea. Brain death at that time had not yet been defined.

The concept of brain stem death

The current operational definition of brain stem death is based on coma, absent brain stem reflexes, and apnoea. This definition has shown functional utility. Medical practitioners and the public continue to become increasingly comfortable with the concept of brain stem death.[9] With brain stem death, there is no response to external stimuli and no spontaneous respiratory activity. In contrast, cerebral death with preservation of brain stem function results in a 'persistent vegetative state'.[10] Aside from the specific needs of clinical transplantation, the concept of brain stem death is important for several reasons:

(1) death of the brain is irreversible
(2) perpetuation of such an irreversible state by artificial means beyond a reasonable period of time serves no useful purpose.

Before making a request for organ donation, healthcare providers must inquire about and address common misunderstandings people have about brain stem death. Healthcare teams should ideally be trained to communicate with the families of patients who may be potential organ donors.[2,11]

The diagnosis

A rapid and accurate diagnosis of brain stem death facilitates the overall organ donor process (Box 3.1).[12] The diagnosis of brain stem death is a clinical diagnosis that must be confirmed by two doctors. Ideally, the

---

Box 3.1 *Criteria for brain stem death*

- A firm diagnosis of the cause of irreversible deep coma and absent brain stem function
- Pupils are fixed, dilated, and unresponsive to light
- The oculocephalic (doll's eyes), oculovestibular (cold water) reflexes are absent. No eye movement should occur during or after slow injection of 20 ml of ice cold water into each external auditory meatus
- There is no response to painful stimulus
- The gag reflex is absent, and there is no response to a suction catheter being placed in the trachea
- No spontaneous respiration occurs in the absence of ventilatory support (apnoea testing)
  - Baseline arterial blood gases are collected. The CO_2 concentrations should be 5.3–6 kPa (40–45 mm Hg)
  - Oxygenate the patient with 100% O_2
  - Disconnect the patient from the ventilator
  - Administer O_2 at 6 l/min via a narrow bore catheter placed in the endotracheal tube
  - Observe the patient for respiratory effort for 10 minutes or until the CO_2 concentration increases to 6.6 kPa (50 mm Hg)

---

consultant in charge and a consultant or senior registrar independent of the first, but not involved with the transplant team, perform two sets of brain stem tests. Both doctors should have appropriate clinical experience, and the results must be accurately timed and recorded in the notes. For the clinical diagnosis of brain stem death, the patient must be deeply comatose and there must be an accurate diagnosis confirming that the coma is the result of irreversible structural brain damage. Conditions of hypothermia (temperature <32°C) and severe glucose, electrolyte (Na^+, K^+, Ca^{++}, Mg^{++}), and acid base abnormalities must be corrected before a final diagnosis of brain stem death is established. Drug overdose should be excluded in particular circumstances.

Apnoea testing is an essential component of the evaluation of brain stem death.[12] Baseline gases must be collected, and the patient should be ventilated with an FiO_2 of 1.0 and normal tidal volume for 10–30 minutes. Mechanical ventilation is then discontinued, and oxygen should be delivered via a T-piece to prevent hypoxia at a flow rate of 6 l/min. The patient is observed for a period of 3–5 minutes (occasionally longer), after which arterial blood gases are drawn. Careful observation for respiratory effort is required. The test is conclusive if the patient remains apnoeic and the PCO_2 reaches 6.65 kPa (50 mm Hg). During the apnoea period, the donor should be monitored continuously with pulse oximetry and electrocardiography.[12]

Brain stem death results in a complete absence of all brain stem activity. The pupils are usually dilated, fixed, and do not respond to light. There is no swallowing or gag reflex. Extraocular activity in response to head turning or cold water irrigation of the ear canal must be absent. During this procedure, the tympanic membrane must be visualised at least on one side and the head flexed to 30%. Spinal reflexes such as a plantar withdrawal, cremasteric, and superficial abdominal responses frequently remain intact but have no bearing on the diagnosis of brain stem death.[13]

Respiratory depressant drugs

Most centrally acting drugs depress respiration and would be expected to influence apnoea testing of brain stem function. However, the pharmacodynamic and pharmacokinetic properties of drugs are altered when patients are critically ill. Drug screens can assist in determining whether respiratory depressant drugs are present, but correct interpretation of the results depends on close liaison between the clinical and laboratory staff. Therefore it is appropriate to avoid termination of life support if any respiratory depressant drug is present.[12]

Pathophysiology of brain death

Insight into the pathophysiology of brain stem death is essential for the optimal management of a potential donor (Figure 3.1). Intracranial

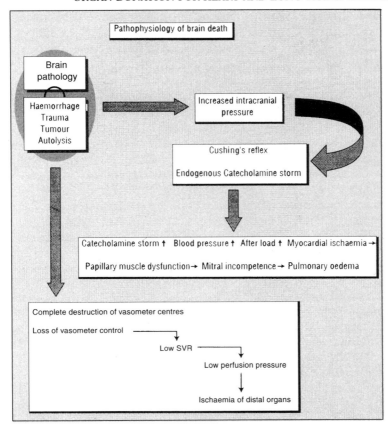

Fig 3.1   The pathophysiology of brain stem death.
This is a schematic representation of the dynamic events following severe brain injury leading to brain stem death and cardiopulmonary dysfunction.

hypertension from whatever cause (usually trauma or intracranial haemorrhage) leads to compression of brain tissue, venous congestion, and secondary changes in the intracranial vessels with destruction of the blood brain barrier. Thus, brain oedema is perpetuated by increased intracranial pressure. A vicious circle ensues, with the intracranial pressure eventually exceeding arterial pressure. Elevated intracranial pressure may then result in transtentorial herniation on the side of a mass lesion, with compression and subsequent herniation of the brain stem into the foramen magnum. As brain swelling continues, all intracranial circulation eventually ceases. When this persists for more than a few minutes, the "no reflow" phenomenon prevents any resumption of intracranial circulation. Autolysis of the brain then ensues.

Cardiovascular changes

An association between acute cardiac dysfunction and intracranial haemorrhage has been recognised for almost a century. Bradycardia and systemic hypertension associated with raised intracranial pressure were reported by Cushing at the turn of the century.

During the acute phase after cerebrovascular accidents, abnormalities of the electrocardiogram are common. Acute subdural haematoma may be accompanied by a variety of arrhythmias, including sinus bradycardia, abnormalities of atrioventricular conduction, supraventricular tachycardia, ventricular tachycardia and fibrillation. Repolarisation changes may be seen on the electrocardiogram with subarachnoid and intracranial haemorrhage including ST segment elevation, T wave inversion, prominent U waves, and QT interval prolongation. Changes on the electrocardiogram, however, do not necessarily imply coronary artery disease in the potential donor.

Diffuse repolarisation changes noted on the electrocardiogram in patients with cerebrovascular accidents have been reproduced by infusion of catecholamines directly into the coronary arteries of experimental animals. Novitzky *et al.* have shown that the haemodynamic effects in a baboon model were secondary to an endogenous "catecholamine storm".[14] A sympathectomy improves the haemodynamic and pathologic abnormalities that are associated with an increased intracranial pressure. Severe brain trauma may result in myocardial injury mediated through the sympathetic nervous system, as suggested by increased creatinine kinase, troponin T and an excess of urinary catecholamines in potential donors.[15,16] Myocardial injury may lead to transient dysfunction of the papillary muscles, resulting in mitral regurgitation, elevated left atrial pressure, and pulmonary oedema.[17,18]

This sequence of events does not occur in all cases of brain injury and is probably modified by the mechanism and the rate of progression of the brain injury as well as other unknown variables.[19] Many haemodynamic abnormalities are usually transient and may even escape clinical detection. Nevertheless, cardiac injury associated with brain stem death may explain why a small number of heart transplant recipients experience unexplained graft dysfunction.[20]

Pulmonary dysfunction with brain death

Pulmonary oedema developing after severe brain injury has been termed neurogenic pulmonary oedema.[19] The exact pathogenesis of neurogenic pulmonary oedema remains controversial because it cannot easily be categorised as either *high pressure* (haemodynamic alterations with pressure or volume overload) or *increased permeability* (alterations of pulmonary capillary permeability) pulmonary oedema. Detailed human studies of neurogenic pulmonary oedema are not available; scattered reports have, however, documented severe systemic hypertension and increases in pulmonary capillary wedge pressures occurring transiently, before the onset of pulmonary oedema. Studies in experimental animals have also shown that severe systemic arterial hypertension precedes the development of neurogenic pulmonary oedema. While the available evidence is inconclusive, primary pulmonary vessel constriction, increased vagal tone, and decreased β adrenergic tone have been implicated in the pathophysiology of high pressure neurogenic pulmonary oedema.[21]

Altered pulmonary microvascular permeability has also been implicated in the pathogenesis of neurogenic pulmonary oedema. Raised concentrations of IL8, a cytokine associated with acute lung injury, have been identified in the bronchoalveolar lavage fluid of donors.[22] The observation of high protein content in the pulmonary oedema fluid and the experimental observation of pulmonary oedema after brain injury in the absence of documented pulmonary microvascular hypertension lend credence to this proposed mechanism. While different mechanisms are likely to be operative in neurogenic pulmonary oedema in various clinical settings, the extreme elevations in systemic arterial, left atrial, and pulmonary venous. pressures noted in experimental models suggest that the hydrostatic abnormalities are the primary factors in neurogenic pulmonary oedema, with permeability defects occurring secondarily. Whatever the underlying mechanism, the final effect of altered capillary permeability results in extravasation of fluid to the intra-alveolar space.

Endocrine and metabolic changes

The neuroendocrine response is a critical component of the adaptive process to trauma, brain injury, and major surgery. The brain nuclei responsible for the neuroendocrine response act mainly by efferent pathways to the hypothalamic pituitary adrenal axis and the sympathoadrenal system. The neuroendocrine response to brain injury is similar to the response observed in patients with extracerebral injury. Generally, there is a biphasic response, with an initial sympathoadrenal storm associated with variable and altered stimulation of the hypothalamic pituitary adrenal axis, followed by endocrine changes including the counterregulatory, gonadal, and thyroid hormones. The outcome after brain injury is closely correlated with the intensity of these hormonal changes.

Experimental studies in animals have suggested that endocrine dysfunction associated with brain stem death leads to a significant depression of cardiac function. Although after the onset of brain stem death the concentrations of many hormones (T3, T4, ACTH, cortisol, insulin) are reduced, cardiac function and circulatory stability can be maintained by volume replacement.[23]

Alterations in thyroid hormone metabolism are recognised after brain stem death. Animal studies show that cardiac function is subject to depletion of high energy phosphates, glycogen, and accumulation of tissue lactate, but the administration of T3 results in reversal of these haemodynamic and metabolic derangements.[24,25] In humans, after brain stem death, although the plasma concentrations of thyroid stimulating hormone remain unchanged, there is a rapid decline in free triiodothyronine levels as well as an elevation of reverse triiodothyronine.[26] There is also evidence to suggest that triiodothyronine receptor density declines, resulting in reduced intracellular triiodothyronine concentrations.[27]

Central diabetes insipidus is seen in 38–87% of brain dead patients. Normally, antidiuretic hormone is synthesised in the supraoptic and paraventricular nuclei in the hypothalamus, transported down the axons of the supraopticohypophyseal tract, and stored in and subsequently released from the posterior lobe of the pituitary (neurohypophysis). Antidiuretic hormone is a prime determinant of renal water excretion; it increases renal water reabsorption by augmenting the water permeability of the cortical and medullary collecting tubules, resulting in increased urine osmolality. In the absence of antidiuretic hormone, water reabsorption is reduced in these segments, resulting in central diabetes insipidus characterised by the production of large quantities of diluted urine, often in excess of 1 l/hr. This massive diuresis may result in severe hypernatraemia, hypokalaemia, and hypomagnesaemia with the attendant risk of cardiac arrhythmias and a reduction in myocardial glycogen content.

Donor management

The importance of management of the cadaver donor is emphasised by the fact that the quality of management of a single donor will ultimately affect the health of as many as eight recipients. Optimal donor management and the prevention of tissue injury after brain stem death potentially reduces the incidence of primary graft failure encountered in organ transplantation.

The organ donor process begins with recognition of a potential donor, usually in an intensive care setting, and ends with completion of the procurement procedures in the operating room. Early recognition of a potential organ donor and referral to the local transplant coordinators helps the donor process by allowing more rapid assessment of donors and prompt institution of donor management practices, thereby increasing the supply of organs in a better state.[2,12]

Minimum criteria for multiorgan donors

The general minimum criteria for multiorgan donors are broad enough to ensure that all potential donors are included (Box 3.2). Potential donors who do not initially seem suitable may, with knowledgeable and careful resuscitation, be perfectly acceptable. All potential donors meeting minimum criteria should be promptly referred to the local transplant coordinator for complete evaluation. The referral process may begin when

---

Box 3.2 *Minimum donor criteria for organ donation*

- Patient meets criteria for brain stem death
- Patient's age is less than 60 years
- Absence of malignancy with metastatic potential
- Absence of sepsis or communicable disease

---

brain stem death is being considered, even before it has been officially declared. Such early referral does not interfere with ongoing care for the patient but allows for preliminary administrative procedures to be initiated. Box 3.3 lists the pertinent donor information that should be relayed to the coordinator during the initial referral. Donor evaluation includes a careful assessment of the social and medical history. This includes details of smoking history, drug abuse, current medications, associated diseases including hypertension, diabetes mellitus, and previous surgery. Those with extracranial malignant disease, acute or chronic infections, or autoimmune diseases should be excluded.

Purulent endotracheal secretions must be Gram-stained and cultured. Sputum, urine, and blood that are culture positive must be interpreted in the context of the clinical circumstances and may or may not preclude organ donation. A chest X–ray film is always obtained to evaluate heart size and to aid the identification of consolidation, atelectasis, and pulmonary oedema.

Each donor should be screened for hepatitis, AIDS, syphilis, and cytomegalovirus. A positive HIV or hepatitis serology excludes organ or tissue donation. Intravenous drug use and haemophilia may preclude organ donation even in the absence of a positive HIV test.

Box 3.3 *Key donor data at referral*

- Name and demographics (age, sex, race)
- Height and weight
- Date of admission
- Cause of death
- Past history
- Social history (smoking, alcohol, risk factors for HIV, drug misuse)
- Clinical events (procedures, cardiac or respiratory arrest, vital signs, electrocardiogram rhythm, haemodynamic status, urine output, ventilatory variables). Drugs (especially vasopressors)
- Laboratory data (ABO blood type, haematocrit, WBC, cardiac and liver enzymes, electrolytes, creatinine, BUN, cultures, urinalysis)
- Declaration of brain stem death
- What the family has been told
- Whether organ donation has been discussed
- Whether consent has been obtained

Laboratory evaluation of the prospective donor consists of biochemical assays for organ specific function, human leukocyte antigen tissue typing, ABO blood grouping, and serologic and microbiologic evaluation for infectious disease. If multiple transfusions have been administered, serologic testing should be performed on blood samples collected before transfusion.

The basic broad criteria based on history and laboratory evaluation apply to all potential organ retrievals. In addition, organ specific criteria must be considered. In cases of multiple organ retrieval, close communication among the various transplant teams is essential because of the different priorities and routines regarding hydration and use of inotropic drugs and vasopressin.

Basic criteria for heart donation includes:

a donor who should be < 55 years of age, with mean arterial systemic pressure of > 60–70 mm Hg, central venous pressure of 6–12 mm Hg, in a patient receiving < 10 microgram/kg/min of dopamine. Q wave and ST elevation on the electrocardiogram exclude donation. Isolated minor ST wave changes do not preclude donation of the heart. In those patients receiving excessive doses of inotropes, hormone therapy and careful titration of ventilatory support and fluid balance may facilitate the reduction of inotropes to acceptable levels.

Basic criteria for lung donation include:

a donor who is < 55 years of age, without significant pulmonary disease, a smoking history of < 20 pack years, a radiograph with at least one normal lung, ventilatory pressure < 30 cm H_2O and a PaO_2/FiO_2 ratio of > 3, for instance a PO_2 > 300 mm Hg (> 40 kPa) for an FiO_2 of 100%. (mm $Hg = kPa \times 7.523$).

Medical management

Medical management of a potential donor entails an immediate and deliberate shift from care aimed at the protection of the injured brain, to therapy directed at satisfying the criteria for organ donation. The principles of medical management include restoration and maintenance of haemodynamic stability and the prompt treatment of complications related to brain stem death.

The most important variable affecting haemodynamic instability in potential donors is circulating blood volume. Many donors have suffered complex injuries that result in hypovolaemia and loss of vasomotor tone. To minimise brain injury, doctors frequently use mannitol and frusemide to reduce intracranial pressure, but at a cost of reducing preload and afterload. These manoeuvres also decrease blood flow to all other organs. Inotropic and pressor agents may have been introduced to maintain haemodynamic stability. Once brain stem death has been declared, restoration of intravascular volume is initiated. Fluid replacement must be undertaken cautiously in order to prevent pulmonary oedema. Three large bore intravenous lines are placed, one of which should be a line to measure central venous pressure. Ideally in some circumstances, a Swan-Ganz catheter may also be placed to optimise fluid management and to titrate inotrope support. A urinary drainage catheter, nasogastric tube, and a radial arterial catheter should be inserted.

The administration of intravenous fluids should be titrated according to the central venous pressure. Often up to 5 l may be necessary to restore the pressure to 6–12 mm Hg, particularly in the presence of polyuria (>300 ml/hr) secondary to diabetes insipidus. In the presence of polyuria a continuous infusion of argipressin at a rate of 0.5–1.5 units per hour is ideal and provides additional inotropic support in a hypotensive donor. Crystalloids with low concentrations of sodium are the preferred form of crystalloid volume expander, as hypernatraemia in the donor is not uncommon. Intravenous fluid composition, however, must be adjusted according to the serum electrolyte abnormalities. A hypotonic saline solution containing dextrose (0.45% dextrose/saline) to preserve intra-hepatic stores of glucose may be administered at a rate of 1 ml/kg/hr in addition to replacing the previous hour's urine output. Transfusions of red blood cells may be administered to raise the haematocrit to approximately 0.3 or 10 g/l.

Early in the evolution of brain stem death, the patient may have severe transient hypertension and tachycardia. Rapid initiation of vasodilator therapy should be considered in order to prevent cardiac subendocardial injury and potentially the subsequent development of pulmonary oedema. The circulating catecholamines may precipitate supraventricular and ventricular arrhythmias, best managed by the administration of potassium supplements, volume resuscitation, and, occasionally, short term intravenous antiarrhythmic therapy. Alternatively, transient bradyarrhythmias may occur in association hypothermia. Such bradycardia, if associated with significant hypotension, may require isoproterenol hydrochloride or epinephrine for therapy. Atropine sulfate is ineffective.

A hypertensive crisis, lasting minutes to hours but almost always transient, may be followed by abrupt loss of vasomotor tone resulting in pronounced hypotension. The loss of tone is thought to coincide with destruction of the pontine and medullary vasomotor structures and terminal loss of all brain stem function. Although careful fluid replacement to normalise haemodynamics is first line therapy, vasoactive agents must sometimes be added.

Dopamine is the preferred inotrope although, as mentioned, an argipressin infusion used for diabetes insipidus also has beneficial pressor effects.[28] If hypotension (systolic blood pressure <100 mm Hg or a mean pressure <70 mm Hg) persists despite adequate volume replacement (central venous pressure of 6–12 mm Hg), dopamine in a dose <10 micro-gram/kg/min is titrated according to systemic pressures (Figure 3.2a). Dobutamine and isoprenaline are not ideal because of their vasodilatory effects, but their use does not preclude donation (Figure 3.2b).[29] Excessive doses of inotropes, particularly noradrenaline and adrenaline, should be avoided in the multiorgan donor because of their potential to increase myocardial oxygen consumption and to disturb regional organ blood flow (Figures 3.2c, 3.2d). Furthermore, catecholamines have been adversely associated with an increase in the incidence of acute tubular necrosis in transplanted kidneys.

A normal serum creatinine and adequate urine output indicates satisfactory renal function. A low urine output (less than 0.5 ml/kg/hr) suggests hypovolaemia, diminished cardiac output, renal disease, or, occasionally, excessive administration of argipressin. If hypovolaemia is corrected and urine output remains low, inotropic support should be initiated. If oliguria persists, as with cardiac resuscitation, a pulmonary artery catheter should be considered to accurately assess ventricular function and volume status, allowing the titration of fluids and inotropic agents to achieve a cardiac index of >2 l/min/m^2 and a systemic vascular resistance (SVR) of 800–1200 dynes/sec/cm^{-5}.

Pulmonary care is aimed at maintaining adequate alveolar ventilation and arterial oxygenation, and preventing atelectasis, infection and pulmonary oedema. Ventilation at tidal volumes of 10–15 ml/kg, with modest amounts (3–5 cm H_2O) of positive end expiratory pressure and an FiO$_2$ titrated to maintaining a PaO$_2$ of approximately 100 mm Hg are recommended. Excessive positive end expiratory pressure should be avoided as it may impair venous return and cardiac output. In contrast, the absence of positive end expiratory pressure may predispose to non-cardiogenic oedema preventing the utilisation of the lungs. High concentrations of inspired oxygen are to be avoided in a potential lung donor. Overhydration must also be avoided because of the risk of precipitating or potentiating pulmonary oedema.[30,31] High concentrations of oxygen are preferred to higher levels of positive end expiratory pressure in donors in whom lung donation is not possible (severe lung contusion) because of the potential adverse effect of positive excessive end expiratory pressure on the cardiac output.

Aspiration, atelectasis, and pneumonia are common in potential donors, and therefore hourly endotracheal suctioning, percussion, turning for postural drainage, and occasional manual lung inflation are critically important. Mucopurulent secretions are frequent in donors with a normal chest x ray film and do not necessarily preclude lung donation. These secretions must be sent for microscopy and culture and the results interpreted according to the clinical circumstances. Flexible bronchoscopy facilitates the evaluation of mucopurulent secretions. At bronchoscopy,

Dopamine infusion conversion chart

Conversion of dopamine in ml/hr to microgram/kg/min. Assuming 200 mg in 50 ml = 4 mg/ml = 4000 microgram/ml

Weight (kg)	1	2	3	4	5	6	7	8	9	10	11	12	13	14
100	0.67	2	2.7	3.4	4	4.7	5.4	6	6.7	7.4	8	8.7	9.4	10
95	0.71	1.4	2.1	2.8	3.6	4.3	4.9	5.7	6.4	7.1	7.8	8.5	9.2	9.9
90	0.74	1.5	2.2	3.0	3.7	4.4	5.2	5.9	6.7	7.4	8.1	8.9	9.6	10
85	0.79	1.6	2.4	3.2	3.9	4.7	5.5	6.3	7.1	7.9	8.7	9.5	10.3	11
80	0.84	1.7	2.5	3.4	4.2	5.0	5.9	6.7	7.6	8.4	9.2	10	10.9	12
75	0.9	1.8	2.7	3.6	4.5	5.4	6.3	7.2	8.1	9	9.9	10.8	11.7	13
70	0.96	1.9	2.9	3.8	4.8	5.8	6.7	7.7	8.6	9.6	10.6	11.5	12.5	13
65	1	2	3	4	5	6	7	8	9	10	11	12	13	14
60	1.1	2.2	3.3	4.4	5.5	6.6	7.7	8.8	9.9	11	12.1	13.2	14.3	15
55	1.2	2.4	3.6	4.8	6	7.2	8.4	9.6	10.8	12	13.2	14.4	15.6	17
50	1.3	2.7	3.9	5.2	6.5	7.8	9.1	10	11.7	13	14.3	15.6	16.9	18
45	1.5	3	4.5	6	7.5	9	11	12	13.5	15	16.5	18	19.5	21
40	1.7	3.4	5.1	6.8	8.5	10	12	14	15.3	17	18.7	20.4	22.1	24
35	1.9	3.8	5.7	7.6	9.5	11	13	15	17	19	21	23	25	27
30	2.2	4.4	6.6	8.8	11	13	15	18	20	22	24	26	29	31
25	2.7	5.4	8.1	11	13	16	19	22	24	27	30	32	35	38
20	3.3	6.6	9.9	13	17	20	23	26	30	33	36	40	43	46
15	4.5	9	14	18	23	27	31	36	40.5	45	49.5	54	58.5	63
10	6.7	13	20	27	33	40	47	54	60	67	73.7	80	87	94
5	13	27	40	54	67	80	94	107	121	134	147	161	174	188

Dopamine (ml/hr)

Fig 3.2a Dopamine infusion conversion chart.
A particular dose of dopamine in microgram/kg/min can be referenced from the weight of the patient (y axis) and the dose of dopamine in ml/hr (x axis), assuming a concentration of 200 mg of dopamine in 50 ml of dilutant.

Dobutamine infusion conversion chart

Conversion of dobutamine in ml/hr to microgram/kg/min. Assuming 250 mg in 50 ml = 5 mg/ml = 5000 microgram/ml

Weight (kg)	1	2	3	4	5	6	7	8	9	10
100	0.83	1.66	2.49	3.32	4.15	4.98	5.81	6.64	7.47	8.3
95	0.87	1.74	2.61	3.48	4.35	5.22	6.09	6.96	7.83	8.7
90	0.92	1.84	2.76	3.68	4.6	5.52	6.44	7.36	8.28	9.2
85	0.98	1.97	2.94	3.92	4.9	5.89	6.86	7.84	8.82	9.8
80	1.0	2	3	4	5	6	7	8	9	10
75	1.1	2.2	3.3	4.4	5.5	6.6	7.7	88	9.9	11
70	1.2	2.4	3.6	4.8	6	7.2	8.4	9.6	10.8	12
65	1.3	2.6	3.9	5.2	6.5	7.8	9.1	10.4	11.7	13
60	1.4	2.8	4.2	5.6	7	8.4	9.8	11.2	1.6	14
55	1.5	3	4.5	6	7.5	9	10.5	12	13.5	15
50	1.7	3.4	5.1	6.8	8.5	10.2	11.9	13.6	15.3	17
45	1.8	3.6	5.4	7.2	9	10.8	12.6	14.4	16.2	18
40	2.1	4.2	6.3	8.4	10.5	12.6	14.7	16.8	18.9	21
35	2.4	4.8	7.2	9.6	12	14.4	16.8	19.2	21.6	24
30	2.8	5.6	8.4	11.2	14	16.8	19.6	22.4	25.2	28
25	3.3	6.6	9.9	13.2	16.5	19.8	23.1	26.4	29.7	33
20	4.2	8.4	12.6	168	21	25.2	29.4	33.6	37.8	42
15	5.5	11	16.5	22	27.5	33	38.5	44	49.5	55
10	8.3	16.6	24.9	33.2	41.5	49.8	58.1	66.4	74.7	83
5	16.6	33.2	49.8	66.4	83	99.6	116.2	133	149	166

Dobutamine (ml/hr)

Fig 3.2b Dobutamine infusion conversion chart.
A particular dose of dobutamine in microgram/kg/min can be referenced from the weight of the patient (y axis) and the dose of dobutamine in ml/hr (x axis), assuming a concentration of 250 mg of dobutamine in 50 ml of dilutant.

Adrenaline infusion conversion chart

Conversion of adrenaline in ml/hr to microgram/kg/min. Assuming 1 mg in 50 ml = 0.02 mg/ml = 20 microgram/ml

Weight (kg)	1	2	3	4	5	6	7	8	9	10
100	0.003	0.006	0.009	0.012	0.015	0.018	0.021	0.024	0.027	0.030
95	0.003	0.006	0.009	0.012	0.015	0.018	0.021	0.024	0.027	0.030
90	0.003	0.006	0.009	0.012	0.015	0.018	0.021	0.024	0.027	0.030
85	0.003	0.006	0.009	0.012	0.015	0.018	0.021	0.024	0.027	0.030
80	0.004	0.008	0.012	0.016	0.020	0.024	0.28	0.032	0.036	0.040
75	0.004	0.008	0.012	0.016	0.020	0.024	0.28	0.032	0.036	0.040
70	0.004	0.008	0.012	0.016	0.020	0.024	0.28	0.032	0.036	0.040
65	0.005	0.010	0.015	0.020	0.025	0.030	0.035	0.040	0.045	0.050
60	0.005	0.010	0.015	0.020	0.025	0.030	0.035	0.040	0.045	0.050
55	0.005	0.010	0.015	0.020	0.025	0.030	0.035	0.040	0.045	0.050
50	0.006	0.012	0.018	0.024	0.030	0.036	0.042	0.048	0.054	0.060
45	0.007	0.014	0.021	0.028	0.035	0.042	0.049	0.056	0.063	0.070
40	0.008	0.016	0.024	0.032	0.040	0.048	0.056	0.064	0.072	0.080
35	0.009	0.018	0.027	0.036	0.045	0.054	0.063	0.072	0.081	0.090
30	0.01	0.02	0.030	0.040	0.050	0.060	0.070	0.08	0.090	0.10
25	0.01	0.02	0.030	0.040	0.050	0.060	0.070	0.08	0.090	0.10
20	0.015	0.03	0.045	0.060	0.075	0.090	0.011	0.12	0.14	0.15
15	0.02	0.04	0.060	0.080	0.1	0.12	0.14	0.16	0.18	0.20
10	0.03	0.06	0.09	0.12	0.15	0.18	0.21	0.24	0.27	0.30
5	0.06	0.12	0.18	0.24	0.30	0.36	0.42	0.48	0.54	0.60

Adrenaline (ml/hr)

Fig 3.2c   Adrenaline infusion conversion chart.
An approximate dose of adrenaline in microgram/kg/min can be referenced from the weight of the patient (y axis) and the dose of adrenaline in ml/hr (x axis), assuming a concentration of 1 mg of adrenaline in 50 ml of dilutant.

Noradrenaline infusion conversion chart

Conversion of noradrenaline in ml/hr to microgram/kg/min. Assuming 4 mg in 50 ml = 0.08 mg/ml = 80 microgram/ml

Weight (kg)	1	2	3	4	5	6	7	8	9	10
100	0.013	0.026	0.039	0.052	0.065	0.078	0.091	0.104	0.117	0.13
95	0.014	0.028	0.042	0.056	0.070	0.084	0.090	0.11	0.13	0.14
90	0.014	0.028	0.042	0.056	0.070	0.084	0.090	0.11	0.13	0.14
85	0.015	0.03	0.045	0.060	0.075	0.090	0.11	0.12	0.14	0.15
80	0.016	0.32	0.048	0.064	0.080	0.096	0.11	0.13	0.14	0.16
75	0.017	0.034	0.051	0.068	0.085	0.10	0.12	0.14	0.15	0.17
70	0.019	0.038	0.06	0.08	0.1	0.11	0.13	0.15	0.17	0.19
65	0.02	0.04	0.06	0.08	0.1	0.12	0.14	0.16	0.18	0.20
60	0.022	0.044	0.066	0.088	0.11	0.13	0.15	0.18	0.20	0.22
55	0.023	0.046	0.069	0.9	0.12	0.14	0.16	0.18	0.21	0.23
50	0.026	0.052	0.080	0.1	0.13	0.16	0.18	0.21	0.23	0.26
45	0.029	0.058	0.09	0.12	0.15	0.17	0.20	0.23	0.26	0.29
40	0.033	0.066	0.100	0.13	0.17	0.20	0.23	0.26	0.30	0.33
35	0.037	0.074	0.11	0.15	0.19	0.22	0.26	0.30	0.33	0.37
30	0.043	0.086	0.13	0.17	0.22	0.26	0.30	0.34	0.39	0.43
25	0.052	0.10	0.16	0.21	0.26	0.31	0.36	0.42	0.47	0.52
20	0.065	0.13	0.20	0.26	0.33	0.39	0.46	0.52	0.59	0.65
15	0.087	0.17	0.26	0.35	0.44	0.52	0.61	0.69	0.78	0.87
10	0.13	0.26	0.39	0.52	0.65	0.78	0.91	1.04	1.17	1.3
5	0.26	0.52	0.78	1.04	1.3	0.16	1.82	2.08	2.34	2.6

Noradrenaline (ml/hr)

Fig 3.2d Noradrenaline infusion conversion chart.
An approximate dose of noradrenaline in microgram/kg/min can be referenced from the weight of the patient (y axis) and the dose of noradrenaline in ml/hr (x axis), assuming a concentration of 4 mg of noradrenaline in 50 ml of dilutant.

extensive bronchitis and secretions emanating from the distal airways point to parenchymal infection, thereby precluding lung donation. In contrast, a normal bronchoscopy in the presence of main airway secretions allows lung transplantation to proceed. Specimens taken at the time of bronchoscopy can facilitate targeted antibiotic therapy in the recipient.

A diagnosis of neurogenic pulmonary oedema is characterised by diffuse, bilateral alveolar shadowing on chest radiographs, arterial hypoxaemia, and mild leukocytosis in the clinical setting of brain stem death. Physical examination typically reveals diffuse crackles in the lungs. It presents most classically within minutes to hours of an acute well-defined insult to the central nervous system.

The prevention and treatment of neurogenic pulmonary oedema in brain dead donors is largely supportive. It entails optimising fluid balance, converting to colloid fluid replacement, the application of positive end expiratory pressure, and diuretic therapy. If high levels of positive end expiratory pressure are necessary to maintain satisfactory arterial oxygenation, a flow directed pulmonary artery catheter should be considered to confirm the diagnosis and facilitate therapy. Neurogenic pulmonary oedema will generally exclude the patient from being a lung or heart and lung donor.

In view of the alterations in thyroid hormone metabolism recognised following brain stem death some teams advise the administration of T3. T3 therapy to unstable donors has resulted in haemodynamic stability, allowing significant reduction of inotropic support. T3 therapy is initiated with a bolus of 4 microgram followed by an infusion of 3–4 microgram/hr. The infusion may be administered as a "hormone cocktail" which includes 20 microgram of T3, 100 units of actrapid, 100 mg dexamethasone made up to 50 ml of 5% dextrose and titrated at 2–10 ml/hr, in conjunction with argipressin if required. After hormone resuscitation, potential heart donors often show excellent haemodynamic function.[32]

Severe brain injury potentially results in hypothalamic dysfunction and a disturbance of thermal regulation.[33] An indwelling oesophageal, rectal, temperature probe should monitor the donor's temperature. Early in the patient's course of illness, hypothermia may occur. Alternatively, progressive hypothermia may be observed, which is further aggravated by the administration of cool intravenous fluids or blood products. Hypothermia contributes to cardiac dysfunction and cardiovascular instability, and core temperatures <30°C predispose to spontaneous ventricular fibrillation. Temperatures <35°C should be corrected aggressively with the use of warmed intravenous fluids and heated blankets.

Most donors will manifest some evidence of a coagulopathy, frequently referred to as disseminated intravascular coagulation, although intravascular coagulation is not usually the underlying problem. The aetiology may well be the systemic release of plasminogen activator from the necrotic brain. If this is pronounced or clinically evident, replacement therapy should be administered to minimise intraoperative loss.

Potential donors are given prophylactic systemic antibiotics, usually a third generation cephalosporin. The empirical nature of this practice seems justified in patients with multiple invasive monitoring lines who additionally have prolonged environmental exposure in the operating room during the retrieval process. Nephrotoxic antibiotics are to be avoided. All potentially contaminated intravascular catheters, such as those placed before hospital admission, should be replaced in a sterile fashion.

Conclusion

The demand for lung and heart transplantation is increasing, but the supply of donors is limited. Strategies for maximising rates of donation and donor utilisation are being piloted. Optimal donor utilisation entails intensive monitoring and careful titration of fluid replacement and inotropic support. These treatment strategies often result in improved survival for six potential recipients of transplants who have life threatening disease.

References

1 Nicholls J, Crombie A, Morgan V, Watson B. Impact of zonal retrieval arrangements in the United Kingdom: the donor coordinator's perspective. *Transplantation Proceedings* 1996;28:142–3.

2 Wight C, Cohen B. Shortage of organs for transplantation. *BMJ* 1996;312:989–90.

3 Hooker A. Donor action: the results of the UK pilot. In: Johnson RWG, ed. *Transplantation '97 Improving organ donation and optimizing outcome*. London: The Royal Society of Medicine 1997:11–17.

4 Matesanz R, Miranda B, Felipe C. Organ procurement in Spain: impact of transplant coordination. *Clin Transplant* 1994;8:281–6.

5 Pollard S. The impact of state legislation on organ donation. In: Johnson RGW, ed. *Transplantation '97. Improving organ donation and optimizing outcome*. London: The Royal Society of Medicine 1997:3–9.

6 Wheeldon DR, Potter CD, Oduro A, Wallwork J, Large SR. Transforming the "unacceptable" donor: outcomes from the adoption of a standardized donor management technique. *J Heart Lung Transplant* 1995;14:734–42.

7 Sundaresan S, Semenkovich J, Ochoa, Richardson G, Trulock EP, Cooper JD *et al*. Successful outcome of lung transplantation is not compromised by the use of marginal donors. *J Thorac Cardiovasc Surg* 1995;109:1075–80.

8 Powner DJ, Ackerman BM, Grenvik A. Medical diagnosis of death in adults: historical contributions to current controversies. *Lancet* 1996;348:1219–23.

9 Cantrill SV. Brain death. *Emerg Med Clinic North America* 1997;15:713–22.

10 Young B, Blume W, Lynch A. Brain death and the persistent vegetative state: similarities and contrasts. *Can J Neuro Science* 1989;16:388–93.

11 Franz HG, DeJong W, Wolfe SM, Nathan H, Payne D, Reitsma W, *et al*. Explaining brain death: a critical feature of the donation process. *J Transplant Coord* 1997;7:14–21.

12 *A code of practice for the diagnosis of brain stem death*. London: The Stationery Office, 1998.

13 Black PM. Conceptual and practical issues in the declaration of death by brain criteria. *Neurosurg Clin North Am* 1991;2:493–501.

14 Novitzky D, Horak A, Cooper DK, Rose AG. Electrocardiographic and histopathologic changes developing during experimental brain death in the baboon. *Transplant Proc* 1989;**21**:2567–9.

15 Kinoshita Y, Okamoto K, Yahata K, Yoshioka T, Sugimoto T, Kawaguchi N, *et al*. Clinical and pathological changes of the heart in brain death maintained with vasopressin and epinephrine. *Path Res Pract* 1990;**186**:173–9.

16 Riou B, Dreux S, Roche S, Arthand M, Goarin JP, Legger P, *et al*. Circulating cardiac troponin T in potential heart transplant donors. *Circulation* 1995;**92**:409–14.

17 Sebening C, Hagl C, Szabo G, Tochtermann U, Strobel G, Schnabel P, *et al*. Cardiocirculatory effects of acutely increased intracranial pressure and subsequent brain death. *Eur J Cardio–Thorac Surg* 1995;**9**:360–72.

18 Bittner HB, Kendall SW, Chen EP, Craig D, Van Trigt P. The effects of brain death on cardiopulmonary hemodynamics and pulmonary blood flow characteristics. *Chest* 1995;**108**:1358–63.

19 Novitzky D. Detrimental effects of brain death on the potential organ donor. *Transplant Proc* 1997;**29**:3770–2.

20 Bittner HB, Kendall SW, Chen EP, Davis RD, Van Trigt P, 3rd. Myocardial performance after graft preservation and subsequent cardiac transplantation from brain-dead donors. *Ann Thorac Surg* 1995;**60**:47–54.

21 Griffith BP, Zenati M. The pulmonary donor. *Clinic Chest Med* 1990;**11**:217–26.

22 Fisher AJ, Donnelly SC, Forty J, Hasan A, Dark JH, Corris PA. Pulmonary inflammation in potential cadaveric lung donors. *Am J Crit Care Med*. 1998;**157**;A327.

23 Hagl C, Szabo G, Sebening C, Tochtermann U, Vahl CF, Sonnerberg K, *et al*. Is the brain death related endocrine dysfunction an indication for hormonal substitution therapy in the early period? *Eur J Med Res* 1997;**2**:437–40.

24 Nilsson B, Berggren H, Ekroth R, *et al*. Glucose–insulin–potassium (GIK) prevents derangement of myocardial metabolism in brain-dead pigs. *Eur J Cardio Thorac Surg* 1994;**8**:442–6.

25 Bittner HB, Kendall SW, Chen EP, Van Trigt P. Endocrine changes and metabolic responses in a validated canine brain death model. *J Crit Care* 1995;**10**:56–63.

26 Novitzky D. Novel actions of thyroid hormone: the role of triiodothyronine in cardiac transplantation. *Thyroid* 1996;**6**:531–6.

27 Montero JA, Malloi J, Alvarez F, Benito P, Concha M, Blanco A. Biochemical hypothyroidism and myocardial damage in organ donors : are they related? *Transplant Proc* 1988;**5**:746–8.

28 Novitzky D. Donor management: state of the art. *Transplant Proc* 1997;**29**:3773–5.

29 Nishimura N, Sugi R. Circulatory support with sympathetic amines in brain death. *Resuscitation* 1984;**12**:25.

30 Pennefather SH, Bullock RE, Dark JH. The effect of fluid therapy on alveolar arterial oxygen gradient in brain-dead organ donors. *Transplantation* 1993;**56**:1418–22.

31 Carlson RW, Scaeffer RC, Michaels SG, Weil MH. Pulmonary edema following intracranial hemorrhage. *Chest* 1979;**75**:731–34.

32 Pickett JA, Wheeldon D, Oduro A. Multi-organ transplantation: donor management. *Curr Opin Anaesth* 1994;**7**:80–3.

33 Reuler JB. Hypothermia: pathophysiology, clinical settings and management. *Ann Intern Med* 1978;**89**:519.

4 Cardiac transplantation

M B Anderson and Stephen Large

Transplantation of the heart has become an established therapeutic option for patients with endstage cardiac disease. Worldwide, there are approximately 3000 heart transplants performed annually. Further growth in the number of procedures is currently limited by the availability of suitable donor organs. As a consequence, the number of patients on waiting lists is steadily growing. This situation has made it increasingly likely that physicians unfamiliar with cardiac transplantation will come into contact with patients either awaiting or having undergone this procedure. The aim of this chapter is to provide a clinically relevant picture of the steps leading up to the operation, the operation itself, and the complex aftercare.

Historical perspective

The history of heart transplantation began in 1905 with Alexis Carrel, a French-born surgeon, who performed the first cardiac transplant in dogs.[1] Transplantation research continued with pioneering work from Medawar who described the process whereby an animal destroyed grafted tissue and termed it "rejection".[2] The era of modern immunosuppressive therapy had begun and with it came clinically succesful kidney transplantation in 1962.[3] In that same year, Lower and Shumway reported the first successful experimental orthotopic cardiac transplant in an animal model.[4] Five years later in December 1967, Barnard performed the first successful orthotopic human heart transplant in South Africa.[5] Several centres worldwide then undertook the operation but the initial results were poor and the procedure temporarily fell out of favour. The discovery of the superior immunosuppressive agent cyclosporin A by Borel in 1976 contributed to the reemergence of heart transplantation.[6] In 1995 there were in excess of 3000 heart and 100 heart-lung transplants performed annually in 257 centres internationally.[7]

Candidates for transplantation

Patients with endstage cardiac disease become eligible for transplantation when the anticipated survival or quality of life is significantly greater following the procedure. Therefore only those patients with severely restricted exercise tolerance and limited life expectancy refractory to other medical or surgical therapies are considered. The ideal candidate for cardiac transplantation has single-organ failure. Patients referred for transplantation undergo comprehensive medical and psychosocial evaluation. Several factors, including active infection, malignancy, severe peripheral or cerebrovascular disease, irreversible renal or hepatic impairment and neurologic impairment need to be carefully evaluated. Heart failure due to dilated cardiomyopathy or ischaemic heart disease remains the most common diagnosis in patients referred for cardiac transplantation.[8] More unusual diagnoses include valvular and congenital heart disease. The results of transplantation are similar regardless of the aetiology of heart failure, with the general exception of restrictive cardiomyopathy due to amyloid infiltration which recurs early in the donor heart.

Assessing prognosis for patients with congestive heart failure is often difficult, but guidelines have been established for determining when transplantation is indicated.[9]

Right heart catheterisation and evaluation of pulmonary artery pressures is required in all patients prior to consideration for transplantation. Elevation of pulmonary vascular resistance (PVR) is associated with an increased risk of death from donor right heart failure following transplantation.[10]

The waiting period

Once patients have completed the pretransplant evaluation and are accepted, they are placed onto the waiting list. Due to the unpredictable availability and overall shortage of donor hearts, this period may be protracted with waiting times occasionally in excess of one year. This time should not be regarded as a static period and patients need to be seen regularly (if only to show they have not been forgotten) and appropriate adjustments made to the medical regimen. In addition, preexisting borderline contraindications to transplantation need to be closely monitored as worsening of these may deny the patient a new heart. Not surprisingly, between 20% and 35% of patients die whilst waiting on lists.[11] This situation worsens as demand continues to increase and donor organ supply to fall.

Deterioration in the patient's condition requires evaluation. Hospitalisation for bedrest and inotrope therapy (catecholamines and/or phosphodiesterase inhibitors) may be required. Where necessary, most centres will resort to temporary mechanical intraaortic balloon pump (IABP) support, to stabilise worsening cardiac failure. If stabilisation is not possible more advanced cardiac support may be considered in the form of left ventricular assist devices. This technology is expensive and complicated by high rates of infection and thromboembolism. Clinical evaluation of this

49

approach continues with early reports suggesting that there may be an improved outcome in carefully selected patients.[12]

A recent analysis of one centre's waiting list showed a peculiar relationship between recipient ABO blood group, height and waiting time to transplantation. Patients carrying blood group O (universal donor) waited the longest and almost twice as long as those with blood groups B or AB. Similarly, tall patients (height greater than 1.76 metres) had significantly longer waiting times.[13]

Donor management

It is estimated that only 15% of all potential donors are currently being utilised for transplantation and the situation is worse for hearts.[14] Transplant donation should be considered and requested in all brainstem-dead patients with preserved cardiopulmonary function. Currently, an upper age limit of 50 is accepted for satisfactory heart donation. Patients receiving an organ from an older donor have a significantly greater risk to life, of similar magnitude to redo heart transplantation.[7] The general criteria for donor suitability are listed in Box 4.1.

In the past several years, based on favourable results obtained with borderline donors,[15,16] donor heart criteria have expanded to meet increasing demand. Brainstem death results in a "catecholamine storm" and the loss of hormonal and vascular homeostasis.[17] This may severely upset the overall haemodynamic picture and lead to the donor heart being inappropriately turned down. Resuscitation is undertaken by administration of vasopressin (antidiuretic hormone) and intravenous colloid. In addition triiodothyronine (T_3) may be given. Crystalloid is kept to a minimum, reducing the opportunity for neurogenic pulmonary oedema to develop.[16] The decision to use a heart is based on the potential for satisfactory function following transplantation. Potter and colleagues described a technique for the functional evaluation of a donor heart by right heart catheterisation.[18] This technique has been shown to expand donor

---

Box 4.1 *Donor criteria*

- Brainstem death declared
- Relatives and coroner's consent obtained
- Age ≤ 50 years
- Negative for hepatitis B, C and HIV
- No significant history of cardiac disease or extracranial malignancy
- No cardiac contusion with major chest trauma
- No systemic infection
- ECG showing no hypertrophy or evidence of infarction
- Haemodynamic stability

---

numbers in the UK by identifying satisfactory hearts previously thought unsuitable.

A further method for maximising available donor organs is through "domino" heart transplantation. Here, patients with endstage lung disease with preserved cardiac function serve as heart donors when undergoing heart-lung transplantation. In addition to increasing the number of potential donors, the technique also has the benefit of shortening organ ischaemic times (every hour of ischaemia adding 10% to the mortality of the procedure).[7] A recent report describes good early and short-term results with the "domino" procedure.[19] Some groups believe that the "domino" heart whose right ventricle has been exposed to elevated pulmonary artery pressures is "preconditioned" for a recipient with a high vascular resistance in the lungs (PVR).

Matching donor heart and recipient

The main criterion for matching donors and recipients is ABO blood group. Other important factors include size matching for height ($\pm 10\%$). Time constraints dictate that crossmatching between donor and recipient lymphocytes be undertaken only when necessary. If a significant reaction has been seen between recipient serum and a standard panel of sera at the time of recipient assessment, a direct lymphocyte crossmatch must be performed before the operation.

It is apparent that survival is impaired when a significant human leucocyte antigen (HLA) mismatch between donor and recipient occurs or when a transplant is performed across ABO boundaries.[20] Crossing ABO barriers is carefully guarded against, but HLA matching is very time consuming and therefore rarely performed.

Donor organs are distributed by allocating appropriately sized population "zones" to each of the nine UK heart transplant centres. This activity is coordinated and monitored by a special health authority, the United Kingdom Transplant Support Service Authority (UKTSSA). It is arguably a fairer method than that of the USA where the United Network for Organ Sharing (UNOS) allocates donor organs according to registered recipient status (whether hospitalised, in intensive care or supported by mechanical device), followed by waiting time on the list and distance of donor from the recipient hospital.

The operation

Organ procurement

Removal of the donor heart is undertaken once the heart has been seen to be acceptable. Cooperation between the heart procurement team and other organ-harvesting groups (kidney, liver, bowel, bone, skin and cornea) is essential to ensure the best outcome for all. The surgical approach is through a median sternotomy. The heart is inspected for regional wall abnormalities, congenital malformations or evidence of coronary artery disease. After all teams have completed dissection, the patient is given a full anticoagulating dose of heparin. The superior vena cava is ligated and divided, taking care to preserve the sinoatrial node. The aorta is crossclamped and cold, high-potassium cardioplegia (St Thomas's 1) infused into the isolated aortic root. Cold saline is poured over the heart in the pericardial cavity, providing topical hypothermia. The heart is freed by division of the inferior vena cava at the diaphragm and the pulmonary veins, arteries, and ascending aorta at their pericardial reflections. The heart is placed in a cold (0°C) sterile storage container for transport. Cold ischaemic times are usually of the order of 3–4 h, though times of 6–8 h have been associated with excellent graft function.

The recipient operation

There are two surgical techniques which are used for clinical heart transplantation, with several variations on each. The majority of procedures (98%) today are orthotopic, where the recipient heart is replaced by that of the donor. At an appropriate time after the donor heart has been examined and deemed appropriate for transplantation by the donor team, the recipient operation is begun. The recipient heart is exposed through a median sternotomy incision. On safe arrival of the donor organ, full cardiopulmonary bypass is instituted using high aortic cannulation and separate superior and inferior vena caval drainage with occlusive snares about them. The patient is systemically cooled (circa 30°C) and the ascending aorta is clamped. The heart is excised at the midatrial level and the aorta and pulmonary arteries are divided just above their valves (Figure 4.1a). The donor heart is prepared by opening up the left atrium through division of all pulmonary veins and the right atrium for the orificice of the IVC towards the appendage along the crista treminalis (Figure 4.1b) If present, a persisting foramen ovale is closed by stitch oversew. Implantation is begun with the left atrial anastomosis of donor to recipient (Figures 4.1c and 4.1d), followed by the right (Figure 4.1e), the pulmonary arteries (Figure 4.1f), and finally the aortae (Figure 4.1g). After all the air has been removed from the heart, the aorta is unclamped and a period of reperfusion allowed before weaning the patient and the new heart from the extracorpóreal circulation.

Heterotopic placement of the donor heart allows the recipient heart to remain and the donor heart to be attached so as to act as a "biventricular" support device (Figure 4.2). This technique has been used extensively by Barnard and colleagues with good results.[21] Factors influencing the choice of the heterotopic technique include significant donor and recipient size mismatch (a small donor heart), pulmonary hypertension and less than satisfactory graft function. This procedure is technically more demanding. The new assist heart lies in the left pleural cavity and there it may compress the middle lobe, compromising pulmonary function and increasing susceptibility to infection. In addition, the heterotopic heart is difficult to biopsy, making the diagnosis of rejection less straightforward. Reduced flow through the poorly functioning or fibrillating recipient heart makes for higher thromboembolic risk. As a result, most centres favour orthotopic procedures.

Following the completion of the procedure, bradycardia is commonly seen due to the effects of cardioplegia and ischaemia on the donor heart. The heart rate can be increased by the infusion of isoprenaline or temporary atrial pacing to maintain an adequate heart rate (circa 100–110 beats per minute). Isoprenaline has the added advantage of acting as a pulmonary vasodilator. Often the pulmonary vascular resistance is high in recipients as a reaction to protracted pulmonary venous hypertension. Reduction by vasodilators has a beneficial effect upon right ventricular function of the donor heart. In the event of significant graft dysfunction and inability to wean from cardiopulmonary bypass, inotropes can be used and

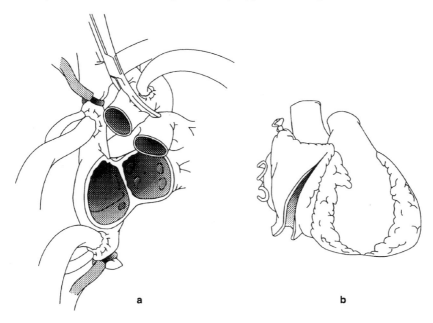

a   b

Fig 4.1   (a) Cardiectomy with prepared aortic pulmonary and artery, left and right atrial cuffs in the cannulated recipient on bypass (aortic return and bicaval venous drainage). (b) The donor heart after excision and preparation for placement within the recipient.

53

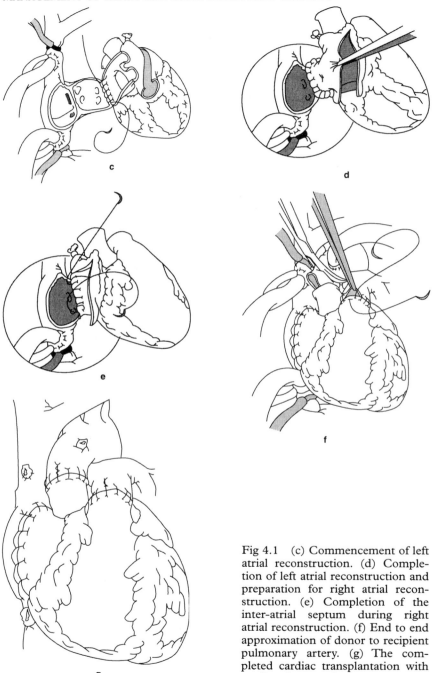

Fig 4.1 (c) Commencement of left atrial reconstruction. (d) Completion of left atrial reconstruction and preparation for right atrial reconstruction. (e) Completion of the inter-atrial septum during right atrial reconstruction. (f) End to end approximation of donor to recipient pulmonary artery. (g) The completed cardiac transplantation with cardiopulmonary bypass removed.

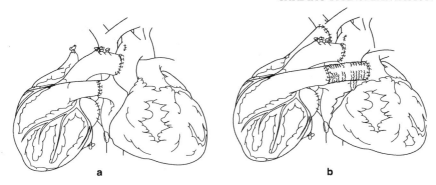

a   b

Fig 4.2   Heterotopic heart transplantation with the donor heart lying in the right pleural space working (a) essentially as a left ventricular assist device (no donor vena caval return but decompression of donor heart coronary blood flow via right side to recipient right atrium through pulmonary artery to right atrial anastomosis), (b) as a bi-ventricular assist with donor to recipient SVC anastomosis, donor PA extended with Dacron interposition graft to recipient PA and left atrial donor-recipient anastomosis and end to side donor aortic to recipient anastomosis).

consideration given to mechanical support. However, primary graft dysfunction following transplantation is uncommon due to advances in donor selection, donor management, and careful matching between donor and recipient.

Immunosuppression

Immunosuppression begins at the start of the recipient operation with the intravenous infusion of 500 mg methylprednisolone. High-dose steroids are accompanied by cyclosporin A, azathioprine and, in some centres, poly- or monoclonal preparations of antilymphocyte globulin. Induction of antithymocyte globulin (ATG) or monoclonal T-cell antibodies (OKT3) may lengthen the interval to the first rejection episode but there is no strong evidence supporting survival benefit.[22] Indeed, there is an increased risk of infectious complications (especially viral) as well as an increased incidence of lymphoproliferative diseases. Over the course of the first two weeks immunosuppression is reduced to maintenance therapy which in most centres consists of "triple therapy": cyclosporin A, azathioprine and corticosteroids. Cyclosporin dosage is adjusted to maintain adequate blood levels whilst observing renal function. Azathioprine is continued at a maintenance dose with attention to white blood cell counts. Long-term therapy is achieved with appropriate reduction of dosages of cyclosporin and prednisolone to achieve a balance between the lowest risk of acute rejection and infection for that particular patient.[23]

Protocols for immunosuppression vary and a list of commonly used agents and their more common side effects is shown in Table 4.1.

Table 4.1   Immunosuppressive medications

Medication	Mode of action	Side effects
Cyclosporin	Blocks secretion of interleukin-2	Hypertension, renal failure, neurotoxicity, hirsutism
Steroids	Lympholytic agent, interferes with antigen recognition	Diabetes, hypertension, osteoporosis, cataracts, obesity
Azathioprine	Purine antimetabolite	Leucopenia, pancreatitis
Methotrexate	Folate analogue, inhibits purine synthesis	Leucopenia, stomatitis
Lympholytic agents (OKT3, antithymocyte globulin)	Opsonises lymphocytes	Allergic reactions, leucopenia, serum sickness

Perioperative complications

This section covers complications seen in the perioperative period, defined here as the day of surgery and the following 30 days. Patients recovering after heart transplantation require at least the same post-operative care as other cardiac surgical patients. However, in addition to the problems seen with cardiac surgery (e.g. relative crystalloid overload, risk of infection and tamponade), transplant patients must be observed for complications specific to transplantation, namely donor heart failure, acute rejection, and infection.

Donor heart failure

Primary graft dysfunction is uncommon in a good donor with ischaemic times even as high as six hours. If the donor was in poor medical condition and required substantial support preoperatively, the myocardial energy stores may be depleted, leading to early graft failure. Inadequate preservation or prolonged ischaemic times can therefore lead to graft failure. There may be unrecognised coronary artery disease resulting in acute on chronic ischaemia. This can be treated with bypass grafting at the time of operation. On rare occasions the recipient may have preformed antibodies to the donor, leading to hyperacute rejection and donor heart failure. Fortunately this is very rare.

In recipients with elevated PVR, acute right heart failure of the graft may occur. Even though the recipient's PVR was within acceptable limits at the time of transplant assessment, it may have insidiously risen during the often protracted wait for an appropriate donor heart or increase temporarily on weaning from cardiopulmonary bypass at the end of the operation. Therapeutic measures for reduction of PVR include the treatment of exacerbating factors (acidosis, hypoxia or hypercarbia) and the administration of pulmonary arterial vasodilators (isoproterenol, nitroprusside, nitroglycerin, prostaglandin E1 or inhaled nitric oxide). In refractory cases, advanced mechanial circulatory support, such as a ventricular assist device or extracorporeal membranous oxygenator support (ECMO), may be necessary.

Acute rejection

The incidence of acute rejection has significantly reduced following the introduction of cyclosporin A, as has the attendant morbidity and mortality. However, most patients will have at least one episode of rejection, most occurring within the first three months.[24] Risk factors associated with acute rejection include female donor–male recipient mismatch, prolonged graft ischaemic time, increased HLA mismatch, previous rejection, and extremes of age. Rejection can cause serious myocardial injury with few clinical symptoms but is usually associated with early signs (Box 4.2).

Significant myocardial dysfunction and congestive heart failure can occur with severe rejection episodes. Routine endocardial biopsies are essential to detect early acute rejection. A standard grading system has been devised to characterise the rejection episode and guide therapy (Table 4.2).

Other non-invasive methods such as ECG tracings or echocardiography are of little use in detecting rejection; however, they have a role in assessing therapy. Mild rejection (cellular infiltrate without necrosis) may resolve spontaneously or require an increase in maintenance therapy. More severe rejection (myocyte necrosis) requires treatment with a pulse of steroids, either orally or intravenously. Failure of response to steroid therapy encourages treatment with antithymocyte globulin. Severe rejection occasionally upsets heart function to such an extent that temporary mechanical circulatory assist may be required. It has been estimted that in 10% of cases rejection is antibody mediated (humoral rejection: myocyte necrosis without cellular infiltration or infection present). Humoral rejection usually responds to plasmapheresis, steroids or cyclophosphamide therapy.

Box 4.2 *Signs and symptoms of acute myocardial rejection*

Symptoms
- Occasionally chest pain
- Oedema and weight gain
- Lethargy and malaise

Signs
- Low-grade fever
- Oedema and weight gain
- Pericardial rubs
- Arrhythmias

Table 4.2   Acute rejection criteria (histological)

Grade	Description
0	No rejection
1	A. Focal (perivascular or interstitial) lymphocytic infiltrate without necrosis
	B. Diffuse but sparse lymphocytic infiltrate without necrosis
2	One focus of aggressive lymphocytic infiltration or myocyte necrosis
3	A. Multifocal lymphocytic infiltrates and myocyte necrosis B. Diffuse lymphocytic infiltration with necrosis
4	Diffuse aggressive lymphocytic infiltrate with oedema, haemorrhage, vasculitis and necrosis

Side effects of immunosuppression

Immunsuppressive drugs may produce significant side effects, resulting in considerable morbidity. Renal dysfunction following transplantation is common and likely to be multifactorial. Influencing factors include preoperative end-organ dysfunction secondary to cardiac failure and heavy diuretic use, the effects of cardiopulmonary bypass, donor heart failure, and renal toxic effects of cyclosporin A. Fortunately, postoperative kidney failure is usually transient. Normally a reduction in the dosage of cyclosporin A is all that is required to restore baseline renal function. However, this increases the risk of acute rejection. In refractory cases temporary haemodialysis may be necessary until renal dysfunction reverses.

Cyclosporin A (CsA) therapy may also be complicated by hypertension, hepatic dysfunction, seizures and, on occasions, gum hyperplasia. Hepatic dysfunction is also seen with azathioprine but its primary side effect is leucopenia. Again, these changes are usually reversible with a reduction in dosage. Polyclonal antithymocyte globulin and OKT3, a monoclonal antibody against T lymphocytes, have adverse effects which include fever, acute pulmonary oedema, and an increased incidence of viral infections and lymphoma (which is more often associated with its chronic use). As a result such therapy is used less frequently.

All immunosuppressive agents increase the risk of infection and this is also true for the steroid preparations. Steroids are also known to result in osteoporosis and varying degrees of diabetes. Up to 10% of patients will require insulin to control elevated blood sugar levels.

Arterial hypertension is common and requires drug treatment in up to 75% of patients. It may be complicated by epileptiform seizures. Hypertension is associated with steroid and CsA therapy and a past history of raised blood pressure.

Infection

Infection is second only to rejection as a cause of morbidity and mortality in the early period after transplantation. Immunosuppression plays a major role in the incidence of postoperative infection. A precarious balance often develops between sufficient immunosuppression to control acute rejection and the consequent risk of infection. Aggressive surveillance and early appropriate antimicrobial treatment are important when signs of infection appear.

Early infection is most commonly bacterial.[25] This is particularly true for patients requiring prolonged invasive monitoring or chest tube placement. Nosocomial, opportunistic infections also emerge during this time, including aspergillosis, legionella and nocardia. Fortunately, the incidence of pneumocystis pneumonia and toxoplasmosis has decreased significantly with the routine use of appropriate prophylaxis. Infective endocarditis in the donor heart remains uncommon.

Although more often seen after the first month, viral infections include Epstein–Barr virus and particularly cytomegalovirus (CMV) and are often donor-acquired infections. The incidence is thought to be greater if an antilymphocyte agent is used as part of the immunosuppressive induction therapy. Patients at particular risk are those who show no serological evidence of past CMV infection and are transplanted with organs from a previously infected individual. The resulting primary infection may be severe but is only rarely life threatening. Matching of donor and recipient for serological CMV status is practised where possible but because of donor shortage and the effectiveness of therapy with ganciclovir, CMV matching has assumed less importance in heart transplantation. The use of CMV-negative blood products can also further reduce the rate of early infection.

Cardiological considerations

Postoperative electrocardiograms are typically abnormal with the most common pattern seen showing a double P wave to every QRS complex, illustrating the presence of recipient and donor sinoatrial nodes. A degree of right bundle branch block is also commonly reported. Characteristically, intracardiac haemodynamics are restrictive immediately following transplant. The elevations in filling pressures usually improve in the ensuing months. In conjunction with this, although functional status (exercise capacity) significantly improves following transplantation, maximal aerobic capacity usually only ever reaches 60–70% of predicted values. Quite why this is so is unknown but denervation of the graft probably has some significant role to play. A blunting of the usual heart rate response to exercise due to reliance on hormonal rather than neuronal triggers is also seen. Vasoregulatory responses are also abnormal. Reinnervation is thought

59

to occur late in about 12% of patients and is associated with an anginal syndrome when transplant coronary disease has been identified.

Results

Perioperative mortality has not changed much over recent years and remains at approximately 9–10%.[8] These results are probably related to pulmonary hypertension, consistently the most common cause of operative death. Most early deaths following the operation are due to infection or acute rejection.

Long-term survival, since the introduction of cyclosporin, has also not changed appreciably. Actuarial survival rates for one, five and 10 years are approximately 80%, 70%, and 50%[8] and are dictated by the emergence of transplant coronary disease. Restoration of a normal life expectancy for patients undergoing heart transplantation will be closer once transplant coronary disease is better understood and, as a result, controlled or abolished.

Conclusion

We wish to leave the reader with the following five salient points.

1. The results of orthotopic cardiac transplantation compare favourably with those of medical treatment for patients with endstage heart disease. Although the number of recipients has increased and patients are living longer, further improvements in results are possible.
2. Immunosuppression still leaves patients vulnerable to fatal infection and malignancy.
3. Transplant coronary artery disease (presumed to be "chronic rejection") is unpredictable in its time of onset and is the major factor limiting long-term survival.
4. Despite attempts to increase the donor pool, there remains a critical shortage of allograft hearts. In this regard, the role of implantable cardiac assist or replacement devices and the development of xenografting techniques remains under evaluation.
5. Future progress in transplantation, including immunology and engineering, will depend largely on the commitment of both science and society.

References

1 Carrel A, Guthrie CC. The transplantation of veins and organs. *Am J Med* 1905;1:1101–3.
2 Medawar PB. Immunologic tolerance. *Nature* 1961 **189**:14–18.
3 Murray JE, Merrill JP, Dammin GJ, Dealy JB, Alexandre GW, Harrison JH. Kidney transplantation in modified recipients. *Ann Surg* 1962;**156**:337–45.

4 Lower RR, Shumay NE. Studies on orthotopic transplantation of the canine heart. *Surg Forum* 1960;**11**:18–25.
5 Barnard CN. The operation. *S Afr Med J* 1967;**41**:1271–6.
6 Borel JF, Feurer C, Gubler HU, Stahelin H. Biological effects of cyclosporin A: a new anti-lymphocytic agent. *Agents Actions* 1976;**6**:648–52.
7 Hosenpud JD, Novick RJ, Breen TJ, Keck B, Daily P. The Registry of the International Society for Heart and Lung Transplantation: twelfth official report. *J Heart Lung Transplant* 1995;**14**:805–15.
8 Kaye MP. The Registry of the International Society for Heart and Lung Transplantation: tenth official report. *J Heart Lung Transplant* 1993;**12**:541–8.
9 Mudge GH, Goldstein S, Addonizio LJ *et al*. Task force 3: recipient guidelines/prioritization. *J Am Coll Cardiol* 1993;**22**:21–31.
10 Murali S, Kormos RL, Uretsky BF *et al*. Preoperative pulmonary hemodynamics and early mortality after orthotopic cardiac transplantation: the Pittsburgh experience. *Am Heart J* 1993;**126**:896–904.
11 The Annual Report of the US Scientific Registry of Transplant Recipients and the Organ Procurement and Transplantation Network: transplant data 1988–1991. Richmond VA: UNOS, 1993.
12 Frazier OH, Macris MP, Duncan JM *et al*. Improved survival after extended bridge to cardiac transplantation. *Ann Thorac Surg* 1994;**57**:1416–22.
13 Sharples L, Roberts M, Parameshwar J, Schofield P, Wallwork J, Large S. Heart transplantation in the United Kingdom: who waits longest and why. *J Heart Lung Transplant* 1995;**14**(2):236–43.
14 Gore SM, Cable DJ, Holland AJ. Organ donation from intensive care units in England and Wales: two years confidential audit of deaths in intensive care. *BMJ* 1992;**304**:349–55.
15 Lammermeier DE, Sweeney MS, Haupt HE *et al*. Use of potentially infected donor hearts for cardiac transplantation. *Ann Thorac Surg* 1990;**55**:222–7.
16 Wheeldon D, Potter C, Oduro A, Wallwork J, Large S. Transforming the "unacceptable" donor: outcomes from the adoption of a standardized donor management technique. *J Heart Lung Transplant* 1995;**14**:734–42.
17 Shivalker B, Van Loon J, Wieland W, Tjondra-Maga,T, Burgers M, Plets C, Flameng W. *et al*. Variable effects of explosive or gradual increase of intracranial pressure on myocardial structure and function. *Circulation* 1993;**87**:230–9.
18 Potter C, Wheeldon D, Wallwork J. Functional assessment and management of heart donors: a rationale for characterization and a guide to therapy. *J Heart Lung Transplant* 1995;**14**:59–65.
19 Oaks T, Aravot D, Dennis C, Wells F, Large S, Wallwork K. Domino heart transplantation: the Papworth experience. *J Heart Lung Transplant* 1994;**13**:433–7.
20 Opelz G, Wujciak T. The influence of HLA compatibility on graft survival after heart transplantation. *N Engl J Med* 1994;**330**:816–19.
21 Novitzky D, Cooper D, Barnard C. The surgical technique of heterotopic heart transplantation. *Ann Thorac Surg* 1983;**36**:476–80.
22 Barr M, Sanchez J, Seche L, Schulman L, Smith C, Rose E. Anti-CD3 monoclonal antibody induction therapy: immunological equivalency with triple-drug therapy in heart transplantation. *Circulation* 1990;**82**:IV-291–4.
23 Radovancevic B, Birovljev S, Frazier O *et al*. Long-term follow-up of cyclosporine treated cardiac transplant recipients. *Transplant Proc* 1990;**22**(3 suppl 1):21–7.
24 Kirklin J, Naftel D, Bourge R *et al*. Rejection after cardiac transplantation: a time-related risk factor analysis. *Circulation* 1992;**86**:II-236–41.
25 Gentry L, Zeluff B. Infection in the cardiac transplant patient. In: Rubin R, Lowell S. eds *Clinical approach to infection in the compromised host*. New York: Plenum, 1987.

5 Choice of procedure and early postoperative management of the lung transplant recipient

J H Dark

Choice of procedure

Introduction and terminology

Lung tissue may be transplanted in various units or subunits, with or without the heart attached. Options include the combined heart and lung transplant and various forms of paired, isolated lungs (i.e. without the heart), variously described as "double-lung", "bilateral-lung" or "sequential-lung" transplant. The third option is the self-explanatory single-lung transplant. Rather more obscure procedures include heart and one lung, single lung with contralateral pneumonectomy, the split-lung approach and lobar transplants, usually from adults to children or adolescents.

The principal factors determining choice include the condition of the recipient's heart, (particularly the left ventricle), the need for a large pulmonary vascular bed, and the state of the proposed residual native lung. Thus, if a "harmless" native lung, particularly if it is free of sepsis, can be left in the contralateral chest, a single-lung transplant can be performed and, indeed, is to be preferred. If this residual lung is not harmless, and particularly if it is infected, a paired transplant is needed.

heart-lung transplant patient

Combined heart and lung transplantation (HLT) was the first procedure to achieve clinical success.[1] It can be applied to virtually all forms of pulmonary or cardiopulmonary disease but is mainly reserved for patients with pulmonary hypertension and particularly for those who really do need both lung and heart replacement. This is best demonstrated by patients with congenital heart disease who have pulmonary hypertension and major intracardiac abnormalities. It is certainly more straightforward to replace the heart as well as the lungs for such individuals although very severe cardiac anomalies have been corrected with concurrent isolated lung transplants.[2] HLT continues to be applied to patients with primary pulmonary vascular disease and normal cardiac anatomy – principally comprising pulmonary hypertension or thromboembolic disease. It is the most straightforward procedure for such patients but, again, if heart-lung blocs are not available good results can be obtained with isolated lung transplantation.[3] It has been very clearly demonstrated that changes in the right ventricle will largely reverse in the face of a near-normal pulmonary vascular bed.[4]

Finally, HLT is still used for patients with normal hearts who require a paired-lung transplant, typically those with cardiac failure.[5] This surgical overkill can be justified if the heart of the recipient is used in another transplant – the "domino" procedure.[6] The operation may be a little more straightforward but the recipient gains a denervated, allografted heart which may develop accelerated coronary disease.

Paired, isolated lung transplants

The logical progression from HLT for patients with pulmonary as opposed to cardiopulmonary disease was the "en bloc double-lung transplant".[7] Clinical experience revealed an unacceptable evidence of tracheal healing problems and also cardiac denervation secondary to the extensive mediastinal dissection.[8,9] The tracheal problem was solved by moving the airway anastomosis closer to the lung parenchyma, either with the "bibronchial"[10] technique or with two sets of hilar anastomoses, the "sequential single-lung"[11] approach. An alternative was to revascularise the recipient's bronchial arteries. This requires a difficult dissection in the donor, is technically demanding, and achieves the same rate of bronchial complications – around 4% – as the best reports of conventional anastomoses.[12]

A logical approach is to use the sequential single or more usually termed "bilateral" transplant for all patients with septic lung disease, many with obstructive lung disease and some with pulmonary hypertension. If both lungs must be removed (the harmful residual lung scenario) or if a large vascular bed is required, this is the procedure of choice.

Most bilateral-lung transplants are performed for cystic fibrosis, bron-chiectasis of other types, and obstructive airways disease if there is a septic element. It is probably preferable to the single-lung transplant for pulmonary vascular disease. There has been a fashion for offering younger patients with COPD, essentially those with α1-antitrypsin deficiency, a bilateral-lung transplant rather than single-lung transplant because of a presumed advantage in terms of functional result.[13] This is not borne out in any comparative studies.

Single-lung transplant

This is the most economical form of pulmonary transplantation. Each donor lung can be placed in a separate recipient. A range of non-infective restrictive and obstructive lung diseases can be treated by single-lung transplant (SLT), principally chronic fibrosing alveolitis and emphysema but also including rarer conditions such as obliterative bronchiolitis and lymphangioleiomyomatosis. Obstructive airways disease is the commonest indication – 35% in the St Louis registry, now superseded by ISHLT (International Society for Heart and Lung Transplantation) Registry, (Box 5.1). SLT may also be performed for pulmonary vascular disease with quite acceptable functional results in the best series.[14] Because of the relatively normal mechanical properties of the contralateral lung, ventilation remains distributed evenly between the two lungs but perfusion is directed almost entirely towards the transplant lung. Reperfusion oedema may be a particularly early problem and these patients can have a very difficult postoperative course. If late airway obstruction develops there is a switch of

---

Box 5.1 *Choice of procedure in lung transplantation*

Single-Lung Transplant:
Restrictive Lung Disease
    Fibrosing Alveolitis
    Silicosis
Obstructive Lung Disease
    Emphysema
    Obliterative Bronchiolitis
    Lymphangioleiomyomatosis
Pulmonary Hypertension
    (If there are reasons to enter only one hemithorax)

Only if the contralateral, native lung is non-septic

Bilateral Lung Transplant:
Septic Lung Disease
    Bronchiectasis, Cystic Fibrosis
    Any of the above with bilateral infections
Obstructive Lung Disease in young patients
Pulmonary Hypertension with repairable/anatomically normal heart *and* normal left ventricle

Heart–Lung Transplant:
Pulmonary Hypertension with irreparable heart
Any of the above with impaired left ventricular function coronary artery disease
Any of the above if the Centre is particularly experienced *and* heart lung blocks are readily available

---

ventilation away from the predominantly perfused transplant lung, resulting in severe VQ mismatch and a massive physiological dead space.[15] For these two reasons, SLT has never gained popularity for pulmonary vascular disease in Europe, particularly as heart-lung blocs are often available.

Special situations (i.e. lobes)

The lung, particularly on the left, divides easily into two separate lobes, with their own airways and vascular supply. These lobes, usually the lower which more normally confirms to the shape and size of a whole lung, can be used as "single lungs" for smaller recipients. Two lobes from one lung, usually the left, can be split to allow the separate lobes to be implanted as a bilateral-lung transplant. In this ingenious approach, the left lower lobe is placed in the left chest and the left upper lobe rotated through 180° and placed on the right.[16] Another approach is to perform bilateral-lung transplant with two lower lobes from living related donors. This was first described by Starnes[17] and he has the largest experience, describing 38 transplants.[18] Most recipients had cystic fibrosis and the donors were usually a family member. Perhaps because the operation, for ethical reasons, was only done when the patient was *in extremis* (often ventilated) and a cadaver lung not available, the one-year survival was no greater than that obtained with unrelated brain-dead donors. Current choice of procedure is summarised in Box 5.1.

Selection of the donor and donor management

Fewer than 20% of brain-dead multiple-organ donors are able to donate lungs. This low figure is the same in North America and the UK.[19] Lungs are unusable because of infection, traumatic damage or poor gas exchange consequent on a variety of other causes of lung injury. It is easy to imagine how a severe brain injury, be it traumatic, vascular or hypoxic, might also affect the lungs. In victims of major trauma there may be direct contusion or the secondary effects of fat embolism or multiple transfusions. The unconscious patient may aspirate but even without this insult, the intubated and ventilated patient is clearly at risk of lower respiratory tract infection. In one survey, 40% of ventilated patients with closed head injuries developed a pneumonia within the first week.[20]

Finally, the state of "brainstem death" is accompanied by further lung dysfunction. Brain-dead patients have increased alveolar capillary permeability, responding with inappropriate increases in alveolar arterial gradient to crystalloid transfusion.[21] In its most extreme form, this is manifest as neurogenic pulmonary oedema. The "catecholamine storm" and an abrupt rise in left atrial pressure which accompanies coning probably causes a sheer injury to the pulmonary endothelium.[22] It is unclear whether this lung injury is reversible in the short term.

Donor criteria

There are two principles of donor selection. An injured lung must not be transplanted, particularly as any preexisting damage will be magnified via ischaemia and reperfusion and may result in poor pulmonary function. Secondly, an infectious load must not be transmitted with the transplanted lung. Infection may be a marker of lung injury, may cause lung injury but, most importantly, may spread unchecked in the lung once placed in an immunocompromised recipient.

To meet these demands, the donor must have reasonably good gas exchange and a clear chest X-ray. In a retrospective study, we demonstrated a correlation between the alveolar arterial gradient in the donor and both early gas exchange and 30-day mortality in the recipient.[23] More recent North American studies showed that some infiltrates and occasionally increased AA gradients were acceptable.[24] Nevertheless, use of suboptimal donor lungs is more likely to result in prolonged ventilation, longer ITU stay, and worse outcome in the recipient. Use of lungs from donors suffering trauma, if other criteria are acceptable, does not increase the risk, although emboli of both brain material and fat have been seen in donor lungs.[25] Older donors, up to the age of 65, can give good outcomes although they are much more likely to have apical bullae (and be prone to subsequent air leak). There is some evidence from international registries that increased donor age is associated with reduced early and late survival.[26] The presence of multiple, different organisms on Gram-stain of the tracheal aspirate implies an intolerable infectious load. Lesser degrees of contamination may be acceptable if other criteria such as chest X-ray, blood gases and length of ventilation are satisfactory. Bronchoalveolar lavage of the donor lung prior to implantation gives useful information about parenchymal (as opposed to upper airway) infection and aids intelligent choice of postoperative antibiotics.[27]

Many of the causes of lung injury are unavoidable, but their effects may be minimised by careful donor management. Crystalloid infusion should be restricted and hypotension, usually from loss of vascular tone, treated with appropriate vasoconstrictors.[28] Chest physiotherapy must be continued after declaration of brainstem death with regular endotracheal suction. Few donors are ideal and the decision to use a lung must be based on a variety of criteria in the donor and consideration of the pathology in the recipient. Any degree of pulmonary hypertension in the recipient is likely to exacerbate preexisting injury of the donor by magnifying the deleterious effects of increased capillary permeability.[29]

Lung retrieval and preservation

Organs are removed via a sternotomy and, in the UK, usually as a heart-lung bloc.[30] If there are separate cardiac and pulmonary teams then sequential removal of the heart and lungs may be the technique of choice.[31]

Lung preservation has been extensively investigated,[32] but the essence is to cool lungs with a solution which will maintain cellular integrity during the ischaemic period. The lungs may be flushed with an intracellular, i.e. hyperkalaemic, crystalloid solution – Euro Collins solution modified by the addition of magnesium[33] – or the colloid Papworth solution[34] and more recently, the University of Wisconsin (UW) Solution.[35] Prostacyclin or one of its analogues is infused into the pulmonary artery before the flushing solution to maximally vasodilate the pulmonary bed and the flow volume delivered at a rate to duplicate the normal pressure in the pulmonary artery. The atrial appendage is opened to allow the effluent to drain out and the lungs ventilated to optimise distribution of the flush solution. When the flushing is complete, and with a crystalloid solution the lungs will be almost white at this stage, the trachea is clamped and divided at full inspiration. A plane is developed between trachea and oesophagus and the heart–lung bloc removed from the mediastinum. This is then packed in sterile bags, as a single unit if heart–lung transplantation is planned or divided into component parts. The heart is removed from the lungs by dividing the pulmonary artery at its bifurcation and then dividing the left atrium to leave a cuff of atrium attached to the pulmonary veins. This is straightforward on the left, where the incision is made midway between the pulmonary veins and the atrioventricular groove. There is less room on the right and the incision runs close to or along the interatrial groove.[30] If the lungs are separated into two, the vascular structures are divided roughly in the midline and there is tissue to spare. The airway is divided by stapling the left main bronchus twice, leaving the trachea attached to the right bronchus. If the right main bronchus is stapled the subsequent division will encroach on the upper lobe orifice and make for a difficult bronchial anastomosis.

Matching of donor and recipient

ABO compatibility is an absolute necessity for transplantation, but there is no advantage to identical ABO matching between donor and recipient. Any tendency, however, to use blood group O donor lungs (the universal donor) for any patient will discriminate against the blood group O recipient (who can only receive O organs) and must be resisted. Blood group O recipients have longer waiting times than others.

Size matching is now usually done on the basis of measured or predicted total lung capacity (TLC) and the measurements made on chest X-ray are now largely obsolete. Type of transplant and diagnosis has an important influence. Paired-lung transplants – Bilateral Lung Transplant, Heart Lung Transplant (BLTX, HLTX) must not be oversized, i.e. the predicted donor's TLC must not exceed measured recipient TLC. On the other hand, oversized single lung transplantation is well tolerated. For patients with emphysema this is rarely a problem because the measured recipient TLC is usually huge and almost any size of donor lung can be accommodated. On the other hand, for patients with fibrotic disease the measured TLC will be inappropriately low and our routine is now to match donor to recipient on height basis (the most important component of predicted TLC).

Matching for cytomegalovirus (CMV) status is pursued to maximise the use of CMV-negative lungs in CMV-negative recipients. If screened blood products are given for such individuals they will virtually never have CMV infections. A large waiting list would allow up to 50% of transplants (the proportion of CMV-negative donors in the population) to be spared subsequent morbidity from CMV. Because of the rarity of previous CMV infection in cystic fibrosis patients, CMV-negative recipients tend to dominate transplant waiting lists.

The recipient procedure

Potential pulmonary transplant recipients are admitted at short notice, often after travelling long distances. On admission, they are rapidly reassessed to ensure they are still fit for transplantation with regard to nutritional state and, in particular, the presence of infection. Other than those with septic lung disease, any patient with a pyrexia or evidence of extrapulmonary infection should have their transplant deferred.

The final decision about the suitability of organs for transplant is made only after visual examination in the donor's chest. To avoid wasting organs (and the effort and expense of the retrieval team), if one lung or, unusually, the heart is not suitable, we usually have a single lung recipient available as a "back-up" patient whenever a bilateral lung or heart-lung transplant is planned.

In the United Kingdom, a system of zonal allocation of organs was introduced in November 1994. Each transplant centre is allocated a zone, usually within driving distance and containing a population proportional to the centre's transplant activity. The centre has automatic use of organs donated in the zone but also an obligation to retrieve and export organs that cannot be used by the centre. These arrangements have increased the interchange of organs and reduced the amount of long-distance retrieval, with considerable cost savings.[36]

Surgical and anaesthetic options

Three different incisions are used for the three principal types of transplant, providing three different anaesthetic problems.

Combined heart-lung transplantation is the most standardised, as full cardiopulmonary bypass is inevitable. Only a single-lumen endotracheal tube is necessary and the incision is usually a median sternotomy. Standard central venous and arterial pressure monitoring is adequate; since the heart is matched to the new lungs, right ventricular dysfunction is unusual and the pulmonary artery catheter is unnecessary. The clamshell incision, with its wonderful access to the pleural spaces, permits a standard heart-lung transplant but if the "domino" procedure is performed (as should be the case in heart-lung transplant recipients with septic lung disease), access to the IVC anastomosis is awkward.

A posterolateral thoracotomy through the sixth interspace is the standard incision for single-lung transplants. Some patients, with pulmonary hypertension or a contralateral pneumonectomy, will automatically need cardiopulmonary bypass. For most of the others it is unnecessary but the decision is made on the basis of haemodynamic tolerance of unilateral pulmonary artery clamping and the ability of the residual native lung to clear carbon dioxide. Much has been written about the difficulty of predicting patients who may need bypass but in practice, we continue to have a pump oxygenator available for every case. We no longer insert pulmonary artery catheters as a routine but continuous end-tidal carbon dioxide monitoring is very useful during the period of one-lung anaesthesia. The single-lung transplant patients are the most precarious from an anaesthetic standpoint. Patients with restrictive disease are usually hypoxic and as a result have pulmonary hypertension, although oxygenation is relatively straightforward once the patient is ventilated.[37] Those with emphysema inevitably suffer a degree of air trapping and, if severe, this can result in mediastinal shift and haemodynamic compromise. There is the ever-present danger of a contralateral pneumothorax when these very fragile lungs are ventilated with positive pressure.

The bilateral-lung transplant reintroduced the clamshell or anterior transverse bilateral thoracotomy incision to cardiothoracic surgeons.[11] Access to the pleural spaces for the removal of the lungs, often the most difficult part of the procedure, is excellent.[38] Separate and sequential removal and implantation of each lung is possible without cardiopulmonary bypass and, indeed, such an approach is the norm in North America.[39] A perfectly placed double-lumen endotracheal tube, for both separate ventilation and prevention of spillage of infected secretions into the new lung, is essential. The haemodynamic state may be precarious, particularly after reperfusion of the first lung following implantation of the second, and careful monitoring with pulmonary artery catheter and often trans-oesophageal echo is essential. The right lung is usually implanted first and has to accept all the pulmonary blood flow during left lung implantation. Particularly during the left-sided pulmonary venous anastomosis, when the heart is lifted and left atrial pressure elevated, intraalveolar oedema often develops on the right. In children and adolescents, too small for satisfactory one-lung anaesthesia, bypass is used routinely and the same approach is taken for live donor lobar transplants.[17] In theory, bypass, with its activation of inflammatory mediators, should be deleterious to the transplanted lungs and such a disadvantage can be demonstrated in laboratory models. However, because of anxiety about haemodynamic instability and reperfusion damage to the "first lung", we have adopted routine bypass for our last 55 bilateral lung transplants.[40] Early function of the transplanted lungs, as assessed by alveolar arterial gradient, is the same as a comparative group of 64 single-lung transplants done without bypass. Bleeding, particularly from division of dense pleural adhesions, can be minimised by the routine use of aprotinin in all these patients.

Specific technical issues

Heart and lung transplant

The key to successful heart and lung transplantation is removal of the old organs without either excessive bleeding or damage to existing structures, particularly nerves. In septic conditions, dense inflammatory adhesions must be divided and this can be particularly difficult at the apex of the chest and behind the hilum through a sternotomy. After freeing adhesions, ideally before heparinisation, the heart is removed first and then the lungs. The phrenic nerves must be protected when the lung hila are freed from the pericardium. The bronchi are usually stapled at hilar level and then the trachea approached through the back of the pericardium, between the superior vena cava and the aorta. The bronchial stumps are brought up into the field, carefully dissecting off mediastinal tissue, controlling haemorrhage from the often enlarged bronchial arteries, and protecting the vagus nerves. Varying degrees of vagal damage have been described anecdotally following heart and lung transplantation and we have documented an incidence of delayed gastric emptying secondary to vagotomy in such patients.[41] Haemostasis is secured meticulously in the posterior mediastinum as this area is completely inaccessible after implantation of the donor heart-lung bloc.

The trachea is divided just above the bifurcation, usually flush with surrounding tissues; extensive mobilisation of the distal trachea is unnecessary. After placing the donor bloc in the chest and passing each lung through paratracheal windows behind the phrenic nerves, the two ends of the trachea are anastomosed end to end, with continuous suture. The aorta, and subsequently the cavae are anastomosed and the organ bloc reperfused.

Single-lung transplant

Most single-lung transplants are currently performed for emphysema and a large deep thoracic incision makes for easy access. However, space can be very restricted in patients with fibrotic lung disease. As soon as the lung is adequately collapsed the pulmonary artery is encircled and then clamped, usually for a trial period of 5–10 min. If carbon dioxide clearance and a stable blood pressure can be maintained on one-lung anaesthesia, a rapid pneumonectomy is performed, ligating vessels outside the pericardium and dividing the bronchus flush with the mediastinum. The pericardium is then opened, to allow creation of an atrial cuff. On the right, it may be necessary to develop the intraatrial groove.

The donor lung is placed in the paravertebral gutter and the bronchial anastomosis performed first. It is important to trim the donor bronchus as short as possible (see below) and achieve an end-to-end anastomosis, avoiding "telescoping". A continuous suture is used across the membranous portion without the interrupted or figure-of-eight sutures around the cartilaginous bronchus. The whole suture line is completely buried in peribronchial tissue. An anastomosis of pulmonary artery and the two venous cuffs is straightforward. Difficulties at these sites occur in less than 2% of patients and are almost completely restricted to small females or those with fibrotic disease, where access may be difficult.[42]

Bilateral-lung transplant

Most patients will have septic lung disease with pleural adhesions and the clamshell incision gives good access when removing the organs. If there are unlikely to be pleural adhesions, a median sternotomy is a very satisfactory approach for a bilateral transplant. Anastomoses of bronchus, pulmonary artery, and atrial cuff are made at each hilum as for the single-lung transplant. It has been our routine to insert both lungs, keeping the first lung cold and bloodless with the pulmonary artery and veins clamped, before reperfusing both simultaneously.

The airway anastomosis

The heart-lung bloc carries a systemic blood supply via coronary-to-bronchial collaterals to the distal trachea. If the two ends of the airway are not devascularised and appropriate tissue apposition is achieved, healing is very reliable. On the other hand, the isolated lung has no systemic blood supply – it is the only solid organ transplanted in this condition. Within the lung parenchyma, the bronchial tree is nourished by pulmonary-to-bronchial collaterals but away from the lung, blood supply to the bronchus is tenuous. Historically, good healing was obtained by wrapping the anastomosis with a vascular pedicle, usually omentum. We have demonstrated that a very low rate of bronchial complication – less than 2% – can be achieved by keeping the donor bronchus very short, i.e. close to the lung

71

parenchyma. It is usual to cut the bronchus *at* the origin of the upper lobe branch on either side. Such an approach obviates the need for any form of wrap. Relatively high doses of preoperative steroids – up to 30 mg od – are also tolerated with this approach.[43]

Reperfusion of the lung

Much of the damage sustained during the period of transplantation occurs at the point of reperfusion. Neutrophil sequestration, followed by free radical activation and the appearance of a variety of inflammatory mediators, occurs during the first 10 min.[44] During this period the vascular endothelium is very sensitive to sheer stress from elevated pulmonary artery pressure. Methylprednisolone 10 mg/kg is given 20–30 min before reperfusion down to the neutrophil response. In the single lung, care is taken to remove the pulmonary artery clamp very gradually as the combination of cold and hyperkalaemia causes tense vasoconstriction in the pulmonary bed of the transplanted lung, although this relaxes within a few minutes. When the transplant has been performed on bypass it is important to increase pulmonary artery flow in a gradual fashion.

Postoperative care

Management of ventilation

Most patients will be transferred to the intensive care unit ventilated with a single-lumen endotracheal tube. The occasional patient undergoing single-lung transplant for emphysema can be extubated on the operating table but this is the exception rather than the rule. The transplant lung is relatively non-compliant with a tendency to alveolar collapse secondary to impaired surfactant function. Ventilation with positive end-expiratory pressure will reduce atelectasis and intraalveolar oedema; with a prolonged expiratory time, it can be applied safely to patients with obstructive airways disease.

The patient can be weaned from the ventilator using criteria applied to standard cardiac surgery patients. When the patient is awake, haemodynamically stable with good gas exchange and no acidosis, and adequate pain control (see later in this chapter), weaning can be achieved with standard techniques.

Many patients with obstructive lung disease, from either emphysema or cystic fibrosis, will be dependent upon hypoxic drive and can only be weaned if oxygen concentration is reduced. These patients can be identified from their preoperative blood gases and even postoperatively from the presence of a continuing compensatory metabolic alkalosis. Hypercapnia is the norm in such patients and an arterial PCO_2 of 9–10 kPa is entirely acceptable during the first few days. One to two weeks may pass before the switch to a more normal respiratory control is achieved.

Primary lung dysfunction

In up to 10% of patients there may be early dysfunction with widespread atelectasis and intraalveolar oedema, amounting in some cases to frank pulmonary oedema. Such fluid is protein rich and represents a transudate through damaged endothelium. This situation may be predicted to an extent by poor function in the donor but is very loosely related to pulmonary artery pressure in the recipient. In a study of the outcome of pairs of single lungs from the same donor given to different recipients, pulmonary artery pressure was a major determinant in the presence of a lung injury picture.[29]

Management of this phenomenon is aimed at maintaining adequate oxygenation by keeping alveoli open and reducing the driving pressure in the pulmonary artery which magnifies the increased permeability of alveolar capillaries. Positive end-expiratory pressure (PEEP) should be used even to very high levels. The patient should be nursed with the transplant lung uppermost, which reduces both venous and pulmonary artery pressure. In patients with obstructive lung disease the poor compliance of the transplant lung may result in mediastinal shift, a process which is amplified by PEEP. Under these circumstances there should be no hesitation in using a double-lumen tube and applying PEEP only to the transplant lung. The non-transplant side is either ventilated at a slow rate with very long expiratory phase or is merely inflated with oxygen. If prolonged ventilation is required, the standard double-lumen endotracheal tube can be replaced with a double-lumen tracheostomy tube (Portex): we have ventilated patients for almost two months in this manner.

Inhaled nitric oxide (NO) is a recent and useful adjunct in the management of these patients. Concentration must be carefully controlled (the range is 5–40 nmol) but there is an immediate improvement in oxygenation (by improving local VQ mismatch) a fall in pulmonary artery pressure and in general a clearing of the chest X-ray appearances. Whilst there are theoretical benefits in terms of improved endothelial function and decrease in neutrophil adhesion, the main benefits of nitric oxide are probably in terms of improved oxygenation and particularly reduced pulmonary artery pressure. There are no randomised prospective trials of nitric oxide in posttransplant lung injury but comparisons with historical controls in a large series suggest a very definite benefit.[45]

Patients undergoing single lung transplantation for pulmonary vascular disease are at particular risk of postoperative lung dysfunction. A preexisting lung injury is magnified by the high pulmonary artery reperfusion pressure, resulting in intraalveolar fluid accumulation and a further reduction in the size of the available pulmonary vascular beds. In the setting of pulmonary hypertension with a hypertrophied right ventricle the pulmonary pressure continues to rise in response to this elevation in vascular resistance, resulting in worsening eodema, intraalveolar haemorrhage and further lung dysfunction. Because the opposite lung has relatively normal ventilatory characteristics there may be a very grave VQ mismatch. Standard management of these patients has been to keep the pulmonary pressure as low as possible with vasodilators, nurse the patient with the transplant side uppermost and maintain deep sedation and paralysis for at least 48 h. By this time any initial lung injury may have recovered and the rises in pulmonary artery pressure seen in the awakened patient are better tolerated. In the best hands these patients can be managed with the same mortality risk as single lung transplants for other diagnoses[14] but in several large series the overall outcome has been less good.

Pain control

The sternotomy is relatively well tolerated and these patients require intravenous opiates for only 24–48 h. Most patients can then be managed on a mixture of oral analgesics. The clamshell incision and, to a lesser extent, the lateral thoracotomy are both very painful and it is now our routine to use a thoracic epidural with a mixture of opiate and local anaesthetic for at least 72 h. Because the patients will often have been on bypass the epidural is inserted the day after surgery, when haemostasis has returned to normal. Good epidural analgesia is established before any attempt is made to wean the patient from the ventilator.

Management of other organ systems

In general, performance of the lung dominates the clinical picture. In the patient with impaired pulmonary function, every effort should be made to contain a state of single-organ as opposed to multi-organ failure. From the haemodynamic standpoint most of these patients have normal hearts and, with appropriate filling pressures, good cardiac output can be maintained without use of inotropes. The exception is the "septic state", probably a Gram-negative endotoxaemia seen after transplantation for cystic fibrosis when cardiopulmonary bypass has been used. Such patients are hypotensive and vasodilated and require vasoconstrictors such as noradrenalin, usually titrated against multiple measurements of cardiac output from a thermodilution pulmonary artery catheter. This stage usually lasts for only 12–24 h but it is important to maintain perfusion of other organs, such as the gut and the kidney, during this period.

A negative fluid balance is encouraged, often with intravenous diuretics, and a striking rise in blood urea and creatinine is seen almost invariably. The patient is catheterised and, although of no proven benefit, low-dose dopamine infusion is usually continued for several days.

Chest drains can be removed as soon as air leak and drainage of blood have ceased.

Mobilisation and early convalescence

In the absence of primary lung dysfunction, stay in an ITU need only be 1–2 days. Even with satisfactory lungs, however, there will be a continued oxygen requirement for some days, a manifestation of impaired capillary permeability and areas of atelectasis. Clearing of secretions, aided by regular and aggressive physiotherapy, is encouraged from the start and pain control is of great importance in this respect.

The urinary catheter is maintained until the epidural analgesia is discontinued. Chest tubes are removed when air leak (usually from lung parenchyma or apical blebs) and fluid drainage have ceased. The patient begins to drink at 36–48 h and will subsequently be encouraged to eat. A previous gastrotomy tube can be used for early postoperative nutrition. There is a large obligatory protein loss during the time of the operation, often in the setting of preoperative malnutrition. Supplemental feeding, i.e. such as fine-bore nasogastric tube, either continuously or overnight, or parenteral nutrition, in selected instances should be instituted whenever there is doubt about normal oral intake.

There has been a progressive fall in early mortality after lung transplantation over the first few years. In the best centres, this now approaches that seen after cardiac or renal transplantation. Careful patient selection, an aggressive attitude toward donor maintenance, and increased experience with the surgical techniques have all contributed to this improvement. However, the most important advance has probably been the gradual progress made by increasing the experienced teams of physicians, surgeons, nurses, and physiotherapists in early postoperative care.

References

1 Reitz BA, Wallwork JL, Hunt SA, Pennock JL, Billingham ME, Oyer PE *et al*. Heart-lung transplantation: Successful therapy for patients with pulmonary vascular disease. *N Eng J Med* 1982;**306**:557–64.
2 Bridges ND, Mallory GB, Huddleston CB, Canter CE, Sweet SC, Spray TL. Lung transplantation in children and young adults with cardiovascular disease. *Ann Thorac Surg* 1995;**59**:813–21.
3 Bando K, Armitage JA, Paradis IL, Keenan RJ, Hardesty RL, Komishi H *et al*. Indications for and results of single, bilateral and heart lung transplantation for pulmonary hypertension. *J Thorac Cardiovasc Surg* 1994;**108**:1056–65.
4 Pasque MK, Trulock EP, Kaiser LR, Cooper JD. Single lung transplantation for pulmonary hypertension: three month haemodynamic follow-up. *Circulation* 1991;**84**:2275–2279.

5 Madden BP, Hodson ME, Tsang V. Intermediate term results of heart-lung transplantation for cystic fibrosis. *Lancet* 1192;**339**:1583–87.

6 Yacoub MH, Banner NR, Khaghani A *et al*. Heart-lung transplantation for cystic fibrosis and subsequent domino heart transplantation. *J Heart Transplant* 1990;**9**:459–67.

7 Patterson GA, Cooper JD, Dark JH *et al*. Experimental and clinical double lung transplantation. *J Thorac Cardiovasc Surg* 1998;**95**:70–75.

8 Patterson GA, Todd TR, Cooper JD, Pearson FG, Winton TL, Maurer J and The Toronto Lung Transplant Group. Airway complications after double lung transplantation. *J Thorac Cardiovasc Surg* 1990;**99**:14–21.

9 Schafers HJ, Waxman MB, Patterson GA, Forst AE, Maurer J, Cooper JD and The Toronto Lung Transplant Group. Cardiac innervation after double lung transplant. *J Thorac Cardiovasc Surg* 1990;**99**:22–6.

10 Noirclerc MJ, Metras D, Vaillant A, Dumon JF, Zimmermann JM, Caamano A, Orsoni PC. Bilateral bronchial anastomosis in double lung and heart lung transplantation. *Eur J Cardiothorac Surg* 1990;**4**:314–17.

11 Pasque MK, Cooper JD, Kaiser LR, Haydock DA, Triantafillou A, Trulock EP. Improved technique for bilateral lung transplantation: rationale and initial clinical experience. *Ann Thorac Surg* 1990;**49**:785–91.

12 Petterson G, Arendrup H, Martensen SA *et al*. An early experience of double lung transplantation with bronchial artery revascularisation using the mammary artery. *Eur J Cardio-thorac Surg* 1984;**8**:520–24.

13 Sundaresan RS, Shivaishi Y, Trulock EP, Marley J, Lynch J, Cooper JD, Patterson GA. Single or bilateral lung transplantation for emphysema? *J Thorac Cardiovasc Surg* 1996;**112**:485–95.

14 Pasque MK, Kaiser LR, Oressler CM *et al*. Single lung transplantation for pulmonary hypertension: technical aspects and immediate haemodynamic results. *J Thorac Cardiovasc Surg* 1992;**103**:475–82.

15 Levine SM, Jenkinson SG, Bryan CL *et al*. Ventilation-perfusion irregularities during graft rejection in patients undergoing single lung transplantation for primary pulmonary hypertension. *Chest* 1992;**101**:401–5.

16 Couteuil JP, Tolan MP, Loulmet DF, Guinvarch A, Chevalier P, Achar A, Birnbaum P, Carpentier A. Pulmonary bipartitioning and lobar transplantation: A new approach to donor organ shortage. *J Thorac Cardiovasc Surg* 1997;**113**:529–37.

17 Starnes VA, Barr ML, Cohen RG. Lobar transplantation: indications, technique and outcome. *J Thorac Cardiovasc Surg* 1994;**108**:403–11.

18 Starnes VA, Barr ML, Cohen RG. Hagen JA, Wells WJ, Horn MV, Scharkel FA. Living-donor lobar lung transplantation experience: intermediate results. *J Thorac Cardiovasc Surg* 1996;**112**:1284–91.

19 *UKTSSA Thoracic Transplantation Audit*. Published by the United Kingdom Transplant Support Service Authority, Bristol, 1996.

20 Hsieh AH-H, Bishop MJ, Kublis PS, Newell DW, Person DJ. Pneumonia following closed head injury. *Am Rev Respir Dis* 1992;**146**:290–94.

21 Pennefather SH, Bullock RE, Dark JH. The effect of fluid therapy on alveolar arterial oxygen gradient in brain-dead organ donors. *Transplantation* 1993;**56**:1418–22.

22 West JB, Mathieu-Costello O. Stress failure of pulmonary capillaries: role in lung and heart disease. *Lancet* 1992;**340**:762–67.

23 Waller DA, Forty J, Corris PA, Gould FK, Hilton CJ, Dark JH. Determinants of early outcome after lung transplantation. *J Heart Lung Transplant* 1995;**14**:394.

24 Sundaresan S, Semenkovich J, Ochoa L, Richardson G, Trulock EP, Cooper JD, Patterson GA. Successful outcome of lung transplantation is not compromised by the use of marginal donor lungs. *J Thorac Cardiovasc Surg* 1995;**109**:1075–80.

25 Waller DA, Thompson AM, Wrightson NW, Gould FK, Corris PA, Hilton CJ, Forty J, Dark JH. Does the mode of donor death influence the early outcome of lung transplantation? A review of lung transplantation from donors involved in major trauma. *J Heart Lung Transplant* 1995;**14**:318–21.

26 Pohl MS, Cooper JD, Patterson GA. The international status of lung transplantation. *J Heart Lung Transplant* 1997;**16**:54.

27 Colquhoun IW, Gascoigne AD, Corris PA, Freeman R, Dark JH. The value of donor lung lavage in the identification of postoperative infection following lung transplantation. *Thorax* 1992;**47**:24–9.
28 Pennefather SH, Bullock RE, Mantle D, Dark JH. Use of low-dose arginine vasopressin to support brain-dead organ donors. *Transplantation* 1995;**59**:58–62.
29 Sommers KE, Griffith BP, Hardesty RL, Keenan RJ. Early lung allograft function in twin recipients from the same donor: kick factor analysis. *Ann Thorac Surg* 1996;**62**:784–90.
30 Kirk AJB, Hilton CJ, Dark JH. Extraction of cardiopulmonary grafts. *Ann Thorac Surg* 1989;**48**:145–46.
31 Todd RE, Goldberg M, Koshal A, Menkis A, Boychuk J, Patterson GA, Cooper JD. Separate extraction of cardiac and pulmonary grafts from a single organ donor. *Ann Thorac Surg* 1989;**46**:356–59.
32 Kirk AJB, Colquhoun IW, Dark JH. Lung preservation: a review of current practice and future directions. *Annals Thorac Surg* 1993;**56**:990–1000.
33 Kirk AJB, Conacher ID, Corris PA, Dark JH. Single flush perfusion using Euro-Collins solution: clinical assessment of early graft function. *Transplantation Proceedings* 1990;**22**:2137–2138.
34 Wallwork J, Janes K, Cavarocchi N *et al.* Distant procurement of organs for clinical heart-lung transplantation using the single flush technique. *Transplantation* 1987;**44**:654–58.
35 Hardesty RL, Aeba R, Armitage JM, Korsos RL, Griffith BP. A clinical trial of University of Wisconsin solution for pulmonary preservation. *J Thorac Cardiovasc Surg* 1993;**105**:660–6.
36 Dark JH, Locke T, Rogers C, Wallwork J on behalf of UK Transplant Support Service Authority. Zonal organ allocation for thoracic organs in the UK. *J Heart Lung Transplant* 1995;**14**:No 1, Part 2, S 38.
37 Conacher ID, Dark JH, Hilton CJ, Corris PA. Isolated lung transplantation for pulmonary fibrosis. *Anaesthesia* 1990;**45**:971–75.
38 Conacher ID, Paes ML. Mixed venous oxygen saturation during lung transplantation. *J Cardioth and Vasc Anesth* 1994;**8**:671–74.
39 Fullerton DA, McIntyre RC, Mitchell MB, Cambell DN, Grover Fl. Lung transplantation with cardiopulmonary bypass exaggerates pulmonary vasomotor dysfunction in the transplanted lung. *J Thorac Cardiovasc Surg* 1995;**109**:212–7.
40 Hasan A, Corris PA, Healy M, Wrightson N, Gascoigne AD, Waller DA *et al.* Bilateral sequential lung transplantation for end stage septic lung disease. *Thorax* 1995;**50**:565–6.
41 Au J, Hawkins T, Venables C, Morritt G, Scott CD, Gascoigne AD *et al.* Upper gastrointestinal dysmotility in heart-lung transplant recipients. *Ann Thorac Surg* 1993;**55**:94–7.
42 Clark SC, Levine AJ, Hasan A, Hilton CJ, Forty J, Dark JH. Vascular complications of lung transplantation. *Ann Thorac Surg* 1996;**61**:1079–82.
43 Wilson IC, Hasan A, Healy M, Villaquiran J, Corris PA, Forty J *et al.* Healing of the bronchus in pulmonary transplantation. *Eur J Cardiothorac Surg* 1996;**10**:521–7.
44 Bhabra MS, Hopkinson DN, Shaw TE, Hooper TL. Critical importance of the first 10 minutes of lung graft reperfusion after hypothermic storage. *Ann Thorac Surg* 1996;**61**:1631–5.
45 Date H, Triantafillow AN, Trulock EP, Pohl MS, Cooper JD, Patterson GA. Inhaled nitric oxide reduces human lung allograft dysfunction. *J Thorac Cardiovasc Surg* 1996;**111**:913–19.

6 Microbiological aspects of heart and heart-lung transplantation

Kate Gould

There is a widely held belief that all patients who have undergone solid-organ transplantation will rapidly succumb to every infection they encounter and that "opportunistic" infections are high on the list of likely aetiologies. As a result, transplant recipients often receive frequent courses of broad-spectrum antimicrobials, sometimes without the benefit of microbiological evidence of infection. In practice, although undoubtedly immunosuppressed, heart and lung transplant recipients are rarely rendered neutropenic and in many cases therapy can be withheld until appropriate specimens have been collected for examination. Similarly, the literature is sprinkled with case reports describing transplant recipients with exotic and unusual infections. In reality, when these patients become infected they usually succumb to the same pathogens as the normal population. Indeed, with the advent of effective prophylaxis regimes, even notorious pathogens such as *Pneumocystis carinii* and cytomegalovirus are becoming less frequently encountered.

There are, however, recognised patterns of infection in transplant recipients which are related to the length of time elapsed since transplantation (Figure 6.1) and steps which can be taken to reduce the incidence of certain types of infection.

The preoperative period

Once a patient has been accepted for transplantation they may have to wait many months before a suitable donor can be found. During this period efforts should be made to bring all outstanding immunisations up to date, including the administration of pneumococcal vaccine and the current

78

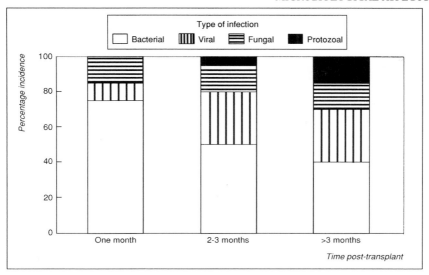

Fig 6.1   Patterns of infection in transplant recipients.

influenza vaccine. Consideration should be given to the use of killed polio vaccine in patients requiring imminent transplantation[1] since the attenuated live strain has been reported to cause invasive disease with paralysis in the immunocompromised.[2] Similarly, in the paediatric population the obvious benefits of receiving mumps, measles and rubella vaccine must be weighed up against a 4–6 week delay in the patient becoming "active" on the transplant waiting list. The requirement for the administration of BCG vaccine pretransplant is controversial and is probably only recommended in areas where there is a higher than average incidence of tuberculosis and when transplantation can be safely postponed for 12 weeks.

Ideally, when a donor organ becomes available the recipient should be in the best condition to receive it. In some centres prophylactic antifungals are commenced as soon as the patient is accepted for transplantation; in our centre we use oral nystatin to reduce the fungal load in the gut and other outstanding issues such as oral hygiene and corrective dentistry should be addressed.

During the waiting time before transplant, genuine intercurrent infection must of course be treated with the most appropriate narrow-spectrum antimicrobial after specimens have been collected for culture. Since transplantation may be delayed until the patient has fully recovered and the antimicrobials stopped for at least 48 h, it is essential that there is good communication between the patient, their local hospital, general practitioner, and the transplant centre in order to avoid disappointment. Information regarding these infections and the microbiology results associated with them can be used to optimise the perioperative antibiotic management plan.

The perioperative period

Individual transplant centres will have their own antimicrobial prophylaxis regimes tailored to the type of transplant and the susceptibility of their local bacterial flora. Patients undergoing lung transplantation for chronic bronchial sepsis present a particular problem to the microbiologist, since both their upper and lower respiratory tract may be colonised with a range of potentially pathogenic bacteria which in some cases, notably those patients with cystic fibrosis, can be panantibiotic resistant. Likewise, the potential for donor-transmitted infection must be minimised. National recommendations regarding the microbiological suitability of donors for solid-organ transplantation have been drawn up and organs from potential donors with evidence of ongoing bacterial infection outside the central nervous system or any confirmed or suspected viral infection should not be used.

All donors are screened for antibodies to human immunodeficiency virus and hepatitis B and C. They are usually also tested for the presence of antibodies against cytomegalovirus at an early stage.[3] This enables transplant centres to match potential recipients to avoid, if possible, implanting organs from a positive donor into a recipient without preexisting antibodies. Unfortunately, there is as yet no standardisation of technologies for cytomegalovirus antibody detection and the rapid latex tests favoured by some centres may result in both false-negative and false-positive results.[4] Although these rapid results are confirmed the following day by more reliable methods, it is too late for heart and lung transplantation where organ deterioration requires implantation within a few hours of retrieval. Since the majority of lung donors will have been mechanically ventilated before the organs are harvested, there is a potential for their airways to become colonised with potentially pathogenic bacteria. Gram stains of bronchial secretions from potential lung donors can therefore provide invaluable information to the transplant centre.[5] Serum specimens from the donor are usually transported back to the transplant centre along with the donor organs and these may provide important information at a later date if the recipient is suspected of suffering from a donor-acquired infection.

The early postoperative period

During this time the recipient can suffer from all the potential infective complications which can befall any patient undergoing open heart or major thoracic surgery. For the majority of heart transplant and single-lung recipients, early extubation and short ITU stay are now the norm and respiratory complications have been minimised. Early atelectasis is frequently encountered in heart transplant recipients and unless the patient is pyrexial or has a significant impairment of lung function, they can be managed with physiotherapy alone without the need for antibiotics.

When an active lower respiratory infection is suspected the range of potential pathogens will depend on a number of factors (Figure 6.2) and the choice of antibiotic therapy will vary accordingly.[6] Access to good respiratory specimens for culture is mandatory since occasionally at this stage posttransplant patients may rapidly succumb to either Gram-negative infections or adult respiratory distress syndrome.[6-9] The inappropriate use of broad-spectrum antibiotics in the latter case will not prevent infection but will predispose to colonisation with more resistant bacteria and fungi at a time when the patient is more vulnerable to infection and will make diagnosis and treatment much more complicated. If preventive measures are necessary, the use of topical agents such as nebulised colomycin or gut decontamination may be more appropriate.

For patients recovering from bilateral-lung transplantation for chronic bronchial sepsis, this period can be the most challenging for the microbiologist for the reasons mentioned previously. Antibiotic therapy has to be juggled carefully to ensure a balance between efficacy against colonising bacteria and selection of panresistant organisms. In those patients previously colonised with *Burkholderia cepacia* or *Stenotrophomonas maltophilia* not sensitive to any antibiotics, early extubation and an effective

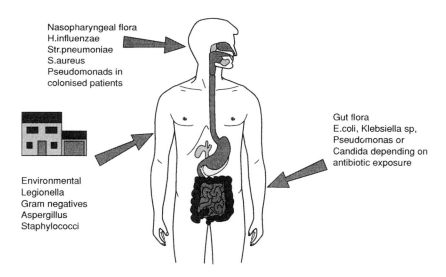

Nasopharyngeal flora
H.influenzae
Str.pneumoniae
S.aureus
Pseudomonads in
colonised patients

Environmental
Legionella
Gram negatives
Aspergillus
Staphylococci

Gut flora
E.coli, Klebsiella sp,
Pseudomonas or
Candida depending on
antibiotic exposure

Fig 6.2   Factors influencing respiratory pathogens

81

pain-free cough is the most effective method of achieving a successful outcome. Indeed, some centres find these organisms so difficult to treat, and the outcome of transplantation so uncertain, that the presence of any of these organisms is a contraindication to transplantation.[10-12]

Urinary tract infections at this stage are infrequent and usually catheter related. For this reason early catheter removal is recommended. Urinary tract infections tend to occur more often in males with a previous history of poor bladder emptying. This group of patients can be identified preoperatively by urinary flow rate and ultrasound residual measurement and urinary tract infections can be minimised by retaining the urinary catheter until the patient can comfortably stand to void.

Wound-associated infections may start to present from about seven days posttransplant. Superficial inflammation can be easily diagnosed and quickly responds to appropriate antibiotics. Deepseated theatre-acquired infections can be more insidious, with the only presenting feature being a rising peripheral white cell count or low-level pyrexia, rarely both, and an apparently normal-looking wound. Blood cultures may be positive in approximately half of all cases. If rejection and all other potential foci of infection have been excluded computerised tomography may be useful in making a diagnosis and guiding the surgeon to the area requiring exploration and drainage. Donor-associated infection can also present in this way. We have had experience of three cases of candida aortitis presenting between two and three weeks postoperatively in patients who received heart-lung blocks from donors whose airways were colonised with *Candida albicans*, in one case despite appropriate antifungals commenced at the time of transplant.

Intravascular line-associated infection may be the source of unexplained pyrexia in this postoperative period and in our experience, an early change of device – not over a guidewire – usually brings about defervescence without sequelae in all patients. Femoral lines carry a high morbidity and should be avoided if an alternative site is available and, if used, must be changed regularly, at least every 48 h. Failure to follow these simple recommendations can result in potentially fatal complications, for example staphylococcal or fungal endocarditis.

The majority of life-threatening infections occurring in the immediate postoperative period are confined to a small group of patients who require a prolonged stay in the ITU, receive augmented immunosuppression for recurrent episodes of rejection or whose renal function precludes the use of cyclosporin and necessitates antithymocyte globulin as an alternative. These patients are highly susceptible to a wide range of nosocomial infections particular to their local environment. For example, some units have a high incidence of aspergillosis, others have small numbers of *Legionella spp.* in their water supply and most transplant units have endemic Gram-negative bacteria and/or methicillin-resistant *Staphylococcus aureus.*

Prior knowledge and experience of the existence of these organisms can guide preemptive therapy as soon as appropriate specimens have been collected. This group of patients may also suffer significant pulmonary infections due to herpes simplex virus presumed to be reactivation of latent infection. Prophylatic aciclovir[13] may be useful in reducing the incidence of this infection but resistant strains are emerging and clinicians must be alert to this possibility in those patients who fail to respond clinically or microbiologically to therapy.

Unexplained fever and neutrophilia in a ventilated transplant patient may also be related to an intraabdominal complication such as pancreatitis or a silent perforation.

One to three months posttransplantation

Assuming there have been no major complications, the majority of heart and lung recipients will have been discharged from hospital by four weeks after transplant. Immunosuppression will still be at a high level, but reducing, and the patients will be beginning to adjust to life posttransplant. It is during this period that cytomegalovirus can become an important cause of morbidity in the transplant recipient.

There is much in the literature about the incidence, investigation, and management of cytomegalovirus in heart and lung transplant recipients and slowly a consensus appears to be emerging.[14,15] Cytomegalovirus can cause a variety of presentations ranging from asymptomatic virus excretion through flu-like illness to life-threatening pneumonitis or gastrointestinal disease. Retinitis is unusual in solid-organ transplant recipients.

Patients who are antibody negative prior to transplant who receive organs from antibody-negative donors and negative screened blood products have a negligible incidence of disease, whereas there is a high incidence in antibody-negative recipients of organs from positive donors and all authors agree that some form of prophylaxis is mandatory in this group.

Currently there are three widely used approaches to cytomegalovirus prophylaxis.[13,15-17] Some groups use intravenous high-titre anti-cytomegalo-virus immunoglobulin given weekly for 6–8 weeks posttransplant or until the patient seroconverts. Alternatively, intravenous ganciclovir can be given for up to six weeks posttransplant or preemptive treatment commenced when significant antigenaemia is detected. Each regime has its advantages and disadvantages. Hyperimmune globulin is expensive and patients often suffer a flu-like illness around the time of seroconversion but it allows the recipient to seroconvert, making troublesome recurrent infection less likely. Ganciclovir is an effective agent but is toxic to both the bone marrow and the reproductive system, particularly in males. Since it is virustatic and not cidal, symptomatic infection may occur when prophylaxis has been discontinued. Preemptive therapy provides the more scientific approach and has been proven to be effective in renal and liver transplantation although these transplant recipients are usually receiving less immunosuppression and cytomegalovirus disease is often more attenuated than in heart and lung transplant recipients. However, it relies on repeated blood sampling and the availability of a reproducible and reliable antigenaemia testing service. This may be impracticable when patients have been discharged from hospital, especially if the transplant centre has a large catchment area.

The role of prophylaxis in antibody-positive recipients is still being debated. With an incidence of disease in this group ranging from 15% to 30%, the potential gains of prophylaxis have to be carefully weighed up against the cost and toxicity of the agents available.

Diagnosis of cytomegalovirus-associated disease can be made by a combination of different methods. The gold standard remains biopsy of the affected organ, when not only can the characteristic inclusion bodies be seen but the level of associated inflammation can be gauged. Excretion of virus in urine and bronchoalveolar lavage fluid can be detected directly by immunofluorescence, by direct early antigen fluorescence on inoculated cell lines, and by culture. Although helpful in making a diagnosis, antibody-positive transplant recipients have been shown to shed large numbers of infected cells asymptomatically. Serology is largely unhelpful; although the appearance of IgM in previously antibody-negative recipients is diagnostic, IgM can persist for a considerable length of time in transplant recipients and it should not be used alone as an indicator of active disease. Detection of antigenaemia has recently found an important place in the investigation of cytomegalovirus disease and in a symptomatic patient from whom biopsies are precluded by underlying disease, a high-level positive test can be diagnostic. However, positive tests in the absence of symptoms or organ dysfunction are well recognised, and if antigenaemia is used as the sole marker for disease, many patients will receive unnecessary treatment. When treatment is indicated, the current mainstay is intravenous ganciclovir but for the reasons mentioned previously, recurrent or relapsing infections in treated patients are not uncommon and adverse effects can be worrisome. Ganciclovir has been shown to be mutagenic in animals and it has not yet been available for long enough to assess the long-term risk of usage in this group of patients who already have an increased susceptibility to malignancy. There can be no doubt, however, that the advent of ganciclovir has improved the outcome in life- or organ-threatening cytomegalovirus disease in solid-organ transplantation.

Primary infection with Epstein–Barr virus will also occur at this time when organs from a positive donor are transplanted into an antibody-negative recipient. In adults this infection is strongly associated with lymphoproliferative[18] disease, so much so that negative recipients are sometimes denied transplantation unless seronegativity in the donor is confirmed. Fortunately, seronegativity in adults is rare and in children, where such mismatches are more frequent, Epstein–Barr related lymphoproliferative disease is much less common.

Three months and beyond

By this stage the transplant recipient should be well established back in the community and, along with their peers, suffer from their fair share of common infections. Generally speaking, they should be managed in the same way with antibiotics withheld unless there is good evidence of a bacterial infection and specimens have been submitted for culture. Recipients with persisting high temperatures, clinical evidence of pneumonia or hypoxia must be referred to hospital for early assessment, which may necessitate early diagnostic intervention in the form of bronchoscopy and bronchoalveolar lavage. Pneumococcal pneumonia is frequently seen posttransplant and if diagnosed and treated quickly, patient morbidity can be significantly improved. Some common viral infections, particularly adenovirus, can cause a devastating illness with permanent sequelae in lung transplant recipients whilst others such as respiratory syncytial virus can be relatively asymptomatic.

Despite the best efforts of the transplant team in the perioperative period, airway colonisation with pseudomonads can persist in patients who have been transplanted for chronic bronchial sepsis. This can be controlled by nebulised antibiotics and the presence of these bacteria in expectorated sputum is not synonymous with active infection caused by them. Indeed, if these patients are admitted to hospital with pyrexia, a new infiltrate on chest X-ray or decrease in lung function, other causes of infection, and particularly rejection, should be sought before antibiotic therapy is commenced since antimicrobial resistance can easily be induced.

Pneumocystis carinii pneumonia is rare before six months posttransplant[19] and is so devastating in lung transplant recipients that most centres now recommend lifelong prophylaxis, whereas in heart transplantation it tends to be used only when augmented immunosuppression is indicated. The most effective anti-pneumocystis prophylaxis is oral co-trimoxazole given for three days each week. Unfortunately some patients are unable to tolerate this and so alternatives such as trimethoprim/dapsone, fansidar or nebulised pentamidine can be substituted. Diagnosis of pneumocystis in heart and lung transplantation is best made by examination of bronchoalveolar lavage fluid with a specific monoclonal antibody. Induced sputum, although helpful in other groups of patients, appears not so discriminatory in transplantation. Again, the gold standard of treatment is high-dose co-trimoxazole, with alternatives such as primaquine plus clindamycin or pentamidine if standard therapy cannot be tolerated.

Other causes of pneumonia such as aspergillosis, nocardia and myco-bacteria must be routinely sought from every transplant recipient presenting with progressive disease, although fortunately these pathogens occur infrequently.

Outcome from fungal pneumonia has historically been poor,[20,21] since these patients often present late and the agent available to treat the condition – amphotericin – is toxic, particularly when used in combination with other nephrotoxic agents as cyclosporin. With the advent of liposomal and colloidal preparations of amphotericin, higher doses can be safely administered at an earlier stage and the prognosis, although still not good, is more hopeful.

Nocardia frequently presents in the chest but has often disseminated and both head and whole-body scan are strongly recommended at an early stage to gauge the extent of the disease. Successful medical treatment, usually with co-trimoxazole, can be curative but may require a lengthy course of treatment.

Primary infection with *Mycobacterium tuberculosis* is uncommon but reactivation of preexisting disease can occur, often at a site distant to the original infection. There is currently a lack of consensus about how to manage patients who undergo transplantation with a good history of previous infection or who originate from a community with a high incidence of tuberculosis. Some centres commence prophylactic isoniazid in all "high-risk" recipients from the time of transplant, others give a full course of therapy, and the rest adopt a "wait and see" approach. Atypical mycobacteria are emerging more slowly as a primary pathogen in organ transplantation than in patients with acquired immunodeficiency syndrome but when they do occur, they are often resistant to many agents, making treatment difficult.

Donor-acquired toxoplasmosis has been problematical in some centres following heart and heart-lung transplantation.[22,23] It is postulated that cysts within the heart muscle reactivate when the organ is transplanted into a recipient without previous exposure to the protozoan and this process is accelerated by immunosuppression. Once reactivated, the cysts set up an acute inflammatory reaction which can present as a pyrexia with cardiac malfunction resembling acute rejection. Diagnosis is usually made by cardiac biopsy, although serology may be helpful in confirming the diagnosis. Toxoplasmosis is unusual in centres which routinely use co-trimoxazole as antipneumocystis prophylaxis, since this agent is also effective against other protozoa.[24]

When the immunocompromised encounter gastrointestinal pathogens, they generally have a higher incidence of infection and their symptoms persist for longer. As a result they may not absorb their medication and are often referred to hospital where blood cultures, if collected, are frequently positive. Despite this, they usually make a complete recovery with appropriate therapy. Rarely, patients may present with acute pseudomembranous colitis, sometimes many weeks following exposure to antibiotics. This is a life-threatening condition and urgent therapy with oral vancomycin and possible surgical intervention is indicated.

In transplant recipients presenting late posttransplant with a low-grade pyrexia and no obvious source, the possibility of malignancy, particularly lymphoma, should be explored. Although this topic will be discussed in more detail in other chapters, some tumours are thought to be Epstein–Barr virus driven and high-dose intravenous aciclovir plays a part in their management. If routinely tested, many solid-organ transplant recipients are found to have extremely high antibody titres (both IgM and IgG) against Epstein–Barr virus. If found in conjunction with malignancy, this is normally entirely coincidental.

Simple fungal skin and nail infections can be particularly troublesome in the transplant recipient. Identifying the pathogen is important since some species have acquired resistance to first-line agents (see below) and since these conditions may be notoriously slow to respond even to appropriate therapy, it may otherwise be some time before a change is initiated.

Attacks of shingles appear to be more frequent in the transplant population, but usually respond favourably to treatment with an appropriate systemic antiviral. Mucosal herpes simplex should be managed in the same manner as in the non-transplant population.

Use of antimicrobials

As mentioned previously, it is tempting to treat all transplant recipients with broad-spectrum, antibiotics at the earliest sign of infection in a well-meaning attempt to stop progression to a life-threatening condition. Indeed, on some occasions transplant recipients have been prescribed agents to prevent them acquiring a spouse's affliction! The logical rules of antimicrobial prescribing should be applied to the transplant and normal population alike but a few additional points should be remembered.

Agents which may interfere with the pharmacodynamics of cyclosporin should, if possible, be avoided. These include all the macrolides (erythromycin and its analogues), tetracyclines, rifampicin, and itraconazole. Synergistic nephrotoxicity can occur with aminoglycosides and vancomycin and these must only be used if antibiotic and cyclosporin levels and renal function can be closely monitored.

Resistant gut flora may have been selected by the use of prophylactic co-trimoxazole, rendering trimethoprim useless for the treatment of urinary tract infection. Similarly, patients whose airways are colonised with *Pseudomonas spp.* have probably been treated previously with quinolones and other organisms may have become resistant to them.

The widespread use of triazole antifungals in hospital and community practice has lead to the emergence of resistant strains, particularly yeasts. As microbiologists, we are attempting to preserve the efficacy of these useful non-toxic agents by encouraging other doctors to confirm their diagnosis mycologically and using topical agents in the management of mucocutaneous candidiasis in the first instance. Reliable sensitivity tests are now available and these should be carried out on non-*Candida albicans* isolates from all invasive infections and those which do not respond to therapy. Some centres' response to the emergency of triazole resistance is to commence systemic amphotericin at the earliest suspicion of fungal infection. Unfortunately this has encouraged the emergence of fungal strains intrinsically resistant to amphotericin and induced resistance in *Candida albicans.*

Other aspects

Paediatric issues

In common with their peers, children who have undergone heart or lung transplantation appear to suffer from one respiratory viral infection after another, but parents become concerned that this is unusual. A small group of patients do go on to get recurrent bacterial chest infections, sometimes requiring prolonged courses of antibiotics before resolution, and the exact mechanism for this remains unknown. Similarly, smaller children may develop persistent problems with postinfective diarrhoea and once the more difficult to irradicate pathogens such as cryptosporidia have been excluded, symptoms resolve when a lactose-free diet is introduced.

Parents are often worried about sending their children to school during epidemics of paediatric infectious diseases such as measles and rubella. With the advent of effective immunisation schedules, these events are becoming far less frequent and the benefit of regular school attendance in this group of children outweighs any potential risk. It is very useful to test all transplant patients for immunity against varicella zoster virus so that in the event of a susceptible individual being exposed, appropriate prophylaxis can be given without delay.

Patient lifestyle

Our environment is littered with potentially infectious hazards for the transplant recipient but with a few sensible precautions, these risks can be minimised.

Dusty atmospheres can contain large numbers of fungal spores and patients should be advised to avoid enclosed areas such as hay barns and animal sheds. Keen gardeners should be similarly warned of the dangers of forking over compost heaps! Pets or stock animals can be kept but patients must not clean cages in areas without adequate ventilation and should, where possible, avoid clearing up after sick animals.

Patients should be warned of the dangers of consuming unpasteurised milk and cheese and swimming in potentially polluted water. Many successful transplant recipients wish to celebrate their new vigour by exploring the world. Most transplant centres produce handbooks listing the potential dangers of foreign travel, particularly in the developing countries, and these warnings must be reinforced when the patients invariably turn to their general practitioner or transplant doctor for immunisation advice. Travel to the more conventional holiday destinations should not be discouraged so long as patients take particular care with food and drinking water.

Immunisation

All live vaccines are contraindicated following transplantation, so alternative killed varieties should be used if available. This precludes travel in all but exceptional circumstances to those countries requiring a yellow fever immunisation certificate (see above). Patients should be advised to have yearly influenza vaccine, although it may not be so immunogenic in this group. Parents with transplants are often worried about the potential risks to themselves when their children receive live vaccines. Although there is indeed a potential risk, it is relatively low since the parent should already have immunity due to either previous exposure or immunisation.

Antibiotic prophylaxis

As microbiologists, we are frequently asked about the requirement for antibiotic prophylaxis to cover various procedures on transplant recipients. Assuming the patient does not have any other predisposing lesion or prosthesis necessitating prophylaxis, once the atrial anastomosis has endothelialised (1–2 months postoperation) the recipient has normal intracardiac blood flow and hence there is no evidence that the heart and/or lung transplant recipient has a greater risk of endocarditis following dental procedures than a normal individual. Prophylaxis for other procedures should follow normal practice guidelines bearing in mind the considerations for choice of antibiotic listed above.

Infection control

In the early days of transplantation, recipients were nursed in isolation, received sterile food, and denied visitors. When they were well enough to leave hospital, they were easy to identify because they had to wear surgical masks in public places! Things have moved on since then but transplant recipients retain their increased susceptibility to hospital-acquired infection throughout their postoperative course and carers have to be particularly vigilant and aware of all potential risks. In Newcastle we have maintained a low incidence of nosocomial infection by adopting a policy of nursing patients in cubicles, with positive pressure ventilation where possible, in the early postoperative period and when they receive augmented immunosuppression. Other centres without access to such facilities manage their patients on open wards.

There are many things to bear in mind. For example, since these patients can often undergo diagnostic or routine endoscopy it must be remembered that additional precautions must be taken with the preendoscopy disinfection procedure, including prolonged exposure times to the disinfectant itself. Building work is almost always taking place somewhere in all hospitals at any time. This work creates dust which will contain large numbers of fungal spores and bacteria such as *Bacillus cereus* from which the patient should be protected a far as possible and very serious consideration should be given to isolating patients receiving augmented immunosuppression.[25]

Many transplant centres have experience of patients with infections due to strains of *Legionella spp* found to be colonising the hospital water supply.[26] Despite the best efforts of the hospital engineers and the microbiologists, this colonisation is notoriously difficult to eradicate and as a consequence extensive and elaborate protocols have to be introduced to protect the high-risk patient.

As a consequence of their immuno-suppression, transplant patients are more susceptible to and require hospitalisation for communicable diseases such as gastroenteritis, varicella and respiratory virus infections. In the acute stages of the illness the patient will be highly infectious, particularly to other immunocompromised individuals, and we prefer to nurse these patients in isolation in areas other than the transplant unit when practicable.

Since the consequences of a simple viral infection can be potentially life threatening to a transplant recipient, especially in the early days posttransplant or when receiving augmented immunosuppression, it makes sense to limit the number of visitors, particularly young children, coming in contact with the patient. Both the patient and their relatives usually appreciate the reasons behind these rules and exceptions must be made for compassionate reasons.

Conclusion

The investigation, management, and prevention of infection in heart and lung transplant recipients provides a particular challenge to the medical microbiologist, particularly with the recent emergence of multiply anti-biotic-resistant and "new" pathogens. It is vital to share experiences with other transplant centres. Since no two centres are environmentally identical and have evolved different patient recruitment and management protocols, direct comparisons between centres should be avoided but it is invariably useful to learn from others' mistakes. In order to fulfil the role effectively, the microbiologist must gain the confidence of surgeons, physicians, paediatricians, general practitioners, and all other health-care personnel. This is probably best achieved by the microbiologist taking an active part in patient management and decision making, even if this entails a 24 h commitment.

References

1 Moore M, Katona P, Kaplan JE, Schonberger LB, Hatch MH. Poliomyelitis in the United States, 1969–81. *J Infect Dis* 1982;**146**(4):558–63.

2 Davis LE, Bodian D, Price D, Butler IJ, Vickers, J. Chronic progressive poliomyelitis secondary to vaccination of an immunodeficient child. *N Engl J Med* 1977;**297**(5):241–5.

3 Petri WA. Infections in heart transplant recipients. *Clin Infect Dis* 1994;**18**:141–8.

4 Freeman R, Gould FK, McMaster A. Discrepant results with a latex agglutination test in the assessment of cytomegalovirus antibody status of cardiac thoracic transplant donors. *Zbl Bakt* 1991;**274**:537–42.

5 Low DE, Kaiser LR, Haydock DA, Trulock E, Cooper JD. The donor lung: infectious and pathological factors affecting outcome in lung transplantations. *J Thorac Cardiovasc Surg* 1993;**106**(4):614–21.

6 Mammana RB, Petersen EA, Fuller JK, Siroky K, Copeland JG. Pulmonary infections in cardiac transplant patients. *Ann Thorac Surg* 1983;**36**(6):700–5.

7 Waser M, Maggiorini M, Luthy A *et al.* Infectious complications in 100 consecutive heart transplant recipients. *Eur J Clin Microbiol Infect Dis* 1994;**13**:12–18.

8 Linder J. Infections as a complication of heart transplantation. *J Heart Transplant* 1988;**7**(5):390–4.

9 Gentry LO, Zeluff BJ. Diagnosis and treatment of infection in cardiac transplant patients. *Surg Clin North Am* 1986;**66**(3):459–65.

10 Scott J, Higenbottam T, Hutter J *et al.* Heart-lung transplantation for cystic fibrosis. *Lancet* 1988;**II**:192–4.

11 Snell GI, de Hoyas A, Krajden M, Winton T, Maurer JR. *Pseudomonas cepacia* in lung transplant recipients with cystic fibrosis. *Chest* 1993;**103**:466–71.

12 Egan JJ, McNeill K, Bookless B *et al.* Post-transplantation survival of cystic fibrosis patients infected with *Pseudomonas cepacia*. *Lancet* 1994;**344**:552.

13 Alivizzatos P, Yavoub MH, Fiddian AP. Oral acyclovir prophylaxis of herpes simplex virus infections after cardiac transplantation. International Acyclovir (Zovirax) Symposium, London, 1983.

14 Maurer JR, Tullis DE, Scavuzzo M, Patterson GA. Cytomegalovirus infection in isolated lung transplantations. *J Heart Lung Transplant* 1991;**10**(5,Pt 1):647–9.

15 Balk AHMM, Weimar W, Rothbarth H *et al.* Passive immunisation against cytomegalovirus in allograft recipients. *Infection 21* 1993;**4**:195–200.

16 Gould FK, Freeman R, Taylor CE *et al.* Prophylaxis and management of cytomegalovirus pneumonitis following pulmonary transplantation – a review of experience in one centre. *J Heart Lung Transplant* 1993;**12**:695–9.

17 Zamora MR, Fullerton DA, Campbell DN *et al* Use of cytomegalovirus (CMV) hyperimmune globulin for prevention of CMV disease in CMV-seropositive lung transplant recipients. *Transplant Proc* 1994;**26**(5, suppl 1):49–51.

18 Gray J, Weghitt TG, Pavel P *et al.* Epstein–Barr virus infection in heart and heart-lung transplant recipients: incidence and clinical impact. *J Heart Lung Transplant* 1995;**14**(4):640–6.

19 Grossi P, Ippoliti GB, Goggi C *et al*. *Pneumocystis carinii* pneumonia in heart transplant recipients *Infection* 21 1993;**2**:75–9.
20 Paya CV. Fungal infections in solid-organ transplantation. *CID* 1993;**16**:677–88.
21 Biggs VJ, Dummer S, Holsinger FC, Lloyd JE, Christman BW. Successful treatment of invasive bronchial aspergillosis after single-lung transplantation. CID 1994;**18**:123–4.
22 Wreghitt TG, Hakim M, Gray JJ *et al*. Toxoplasmosis in heart and heart and lung transplant recipients. *J Clin Pathol* 1989;**42**:194–9.
23 Speirs GE, Hakim M, Calne RY, Wreghitt TG. Relative risk of donor-transmitted *Toxoplasma gondii* infection in heart, liver and kidney transplant recipients. *Clin Transplant* 1988;**2**:257–60.
24 Orr KE, Gould FK, Short G *et al*. Outcome of *Toxoplasma gondii* mismatches in heart transplant recipients over a period of 8 years. *J Infect* 1994;**29**:249–53.
25 Beyer J, Schwartz S, Heinemann V, Siegert W. Strategies in prevention of invasive pulmonary aspergillosis in immunosuppressed or neutropenic patients. *Antimicrob Agents Chemother* 1994;**38**(5):911–17.
26 Parry MF, Stampleman L, Hutchinson JH *et al*. Waterborne *Legionella bozemanii* and nosocomial pneumonia in immunosuppressed patients. *Ann Intern Med* 1985;**103**:205–10.

7 Histopathology of heart and lung transplantation

Susan Stewart and NRB Cary

Introduction

The histopathology of heart and lung transplantation is now well described and established as an essential component of the management of these patients. The biopsy workload soon becomes a significant commitment as a thoracic transplant programme progresses, often pivotal to the patient's treatment. This chapter aims to present both an overview and sufficient detail to guide histopathologists in this important field. We stress the need for specialist histopathologist support within a multidisciplinary setting and highlight areas of particular practical difficulty.

The pathology of the excised heart

Orthotopic heart transplantation has become an established treatment for endstage cardiac failure.[1] Heterotopic transplantation is generally a less satisfactory procedure which is only used in certain specific circumstances. The International Society for Heart-Lung Transplantation (ISHLT) registry figures for 1996[2] record 34 326 heart transplantations worldwide from 271 centres and 1954 combined heart-lung transplantations from 105 centres since the registry began in 1982.

The pathology of the excised heart reflects the causes of endstage cardiac failure, principally ischaemic heart disease and dilated cardiomyopathy, with the latter group being somewhat younger than the former. Other cardiac pathologies may on occasion be transplanted. Pathological examination of the excised heart needs to be carefully coordinated with the harvesting of material for research purposes, given the very valuable resource that freshly excised cardiac tissue represents. It is important to confirm the pretransplant diagnosis and to exclude other unsuspected novel or additional pathologies. This is particularly important in the case of cardiomyopathies, as endstage ischaemic heart disease has generally been well established through detailed cardiac physiological studies and coronary

93

angiography. In fact, as the latter is generally superior to histology in terms of assessing coronary artery disease, examination of the coronary arterial system histologically only needs to be minimal. The same applies to examination of valvular tissue in endstage valvular heart disease where diseased valves will often have been excised and replaced by prostheses many years previously. The key element in histological examination is ventricular myocardial sampling. This allows not only confirmation of distribution of scarring in ischaemic heart disease but also adequate examination of tissue for exclusion of disease processes such as amyloidosis and cardiac sarcoidosis in cases which may have been diagnosed simply as dilated cardiomyopathy prior to transplant. Myocardial histology adds little, however, to most cases of dilated cardiomyopathy, revealing simply variation in myocyte size with variable degrees of myocardial fibrosis. Myocardial histology may, however, show other unexpected features. In some cases of otherwise unequivocal endstage ischaemic heart disease there may be florid myocardial infiltration by eosinophils[3] and this is thought to be a manifestation of drug hypersensitivity, probably a reflection of polypharmacy which is often the case in severe heart failure.

Those with severe heart failure who would potentially benefit from transplantation far outweigh the number of organs available for transplant and consequently strict rationing criteria are adopted by most transplant centres with death on the waiting list an unavoidably frequent phenomenon. After transplantation some early deaths are still to be expected due to failure of adequate function of the donor organ and there are multifactorial reasons for this. Early deaths due to rejection or infection, though still seen occasionally, are largely a feature of the past. This is not only due to more effective immunosuppressive regimes but also a reflection of improvements in the treatment of rejection through adherence to biopsy protocols and histopathological grading of rejection. Long-term survival is still limited by the development of chronic rejection principally manifested as coronary graft vascular disease.[4]

The pathology of the excised lung(s)

There is broad clinical agreement on matching combined, single- or double-lung transplantation to the underlying recipient diagnosis.[2] In endstage combined cardiopulmonary disease where the native heart will not recover, a combined graft is indicated and where there is pulmonary sepsis (e.g. bronchiectasis, cystic fibrosis) both lungs must be removed. Chronic obstructive airways disease and pulmonary fibrosis can be successfully treated by single-lung transplantation. In practice, the three main indications for combined heart-lung transplantation are congenital heart disease, pulmonary hypertension, and cystic fibrosis. The number of heart-lung transplants peaked in 1989, declining because of increased use

Table 7.1   Final pathological diagnosis in 183 explanted lungs[5]

Cystic fibrosis	66
Emphysema	59
Pulmonary fibrosis	19
Bronchiectasis	17
Sarcoidosis	10
Langerhans cell histiocytosis	3
Pulmonary venoocclusive disease	3
Posttransplant OB	2
Rheumatoid OB	1
Haemosiderosis–primary	1
Extrinsic allergic alveolitis	1
Pneumoconiosis	1

of single- and double-lung grafts. Further growth in the total number of cardiothoracic transplants is now severely limited by suitable donor supply. Patients referred for combined or isolated lung transplants for parenchymal disease frequently have clinical and radiological-based diagnoses with limited or no previous biopsy material available. It may be inappropriate to attempt to obtain tissue late in the course of a progressive disease where specific features are unlikely to be present. A histopathological review of 183 explanted lungs over a 10-year period revealed a significant discrepancy between referral and explant histopathological diagnoses and provided guidelines for the preoperative assessment of future recipients.[5] The final pathological diagnoses are shown in Table 7.1 and unsuspected diagnoses in Tables 7.2 and 7.3. Four cases of active tuberculosis were hitherto unsuspected in single-lung recipients who required postoperative antituberculous chemotherapy in view of the remaining native lung,

Table 7.2   Novel and unsuspected diagnoses in lung explants from 17 heart-lung recipients[5]

Referral diagnosis		Final pathological diagnosis	
Cystic fibrosis	5	Cystic fibrosis + Aspergillus	2
		Cystic fibrosis + BCG	3
Bronchiectasis	5	Venoocclusive disease	2
		+ old tuberculosis	1
		+ aspiration	1
		+ bronchocentric granulomatosis	1
Pulmonary fibrosis	4	Sarcoidosis	3
		+ carcinoma of lung	1
Emphysema	2	+ old tuberculosis	1
		+ sarcoidosis	1
Sarcoidosis	1	Pulmonary fibrosis and hypertensive changes	1

BCG, bronchocentric granulomatosis
+, additional diagnosis

Table 7.3 Novel and unsuspected diagnoses in lung explants from 12 single-lung recipients[5]

Referral diagnosis		Final pathological diagnosis	
Emphysema	6	+ TB AFB +ve	3
		+ TB AFB −ve	2
		+ sarcoidosis	1
Pulmonary fibrosis	3	Sarcoidosis	3
Sarcoidosis	2	Pulmonary fibrosis with AFB +ve TB, aspergilloma	1
		Venooclusive disease	1
Bronchiectasis*	1	+ sarcoidosis	1

* Patient intended to undergo bilateral lung transplantation but died intraoperatively.
TB, tuberculosis
AFB, acid-fast bacilli
+, additional diagnosis

complicating their immunosuppressive regimes. Four further cases of unsuspected tuberculosis were identified together with nine cases of sarcoidosis, six of which were unsuspected primary diagnoses and three were additional diagnoses. Sarcoidosis is known to recur in the grafted lung and although this has not been clinically significant so far, the presence of frequent non-caseating granulomas in posttransplant biopsy material requires accurate knowledge of the explant diagnosis for correct interpretation.[6,7] Two cases of aspergillus infection and three of bronchocentric granulomatosis were identified in cystic fibrosis patients, one of whom died of invasive aspergillosis postoperatively which spread from a residual pleural focus. The discrepancy rate was 19% in single lungs and 16% in heart-lung recipients for clinically significant and novel and unsuspected diagnoses. From this study improvements have been suggested in the investigation and management of patients with endstage pulmonary disease who may be referred for transplantation, emphasising the importance of accurate tissue diagnosis in single-lung recipients where a diseased native lung remains *in situ*.

A recent case of misdiagnosed pulmonary lymphangioleiomyomatosis treated with single-lung transplantation who actually had metastatic low-grade endometrial sarcoma highlights the importance of accurate preoperative diagnosis and review of previous material.

Pathology and grading of acute rejection in the heart

In spite of the development of an enormous variety of methods for monitoring rejection in the heart, the right ventricular endomyocardial biopsy as described by Caves[8] remains the method of choice. Histopathological examination focuses on cellular infiltrates with grading systems in general terms taking account of both distribution and intensity as well as myocardial damage. Whilst this approach appears to concentrate on cellular rejection, humoral phenomena are also likely to be important. However, it must be remembered that most significant humoral immune mechanisms are likely ultimately to give rise to cellular infiltrates, e.g. attraction of macrophages in areas of damage or through the Fc receptor of bound antibody. Furthermore, grading systems that rely entirely on cellular infiltrates are well proven over many years. Some centres, however, attempt to identify humoral rejection mechanisms in isolation, advocating staining for complement and antibodies in biopsy material.[9] Reports in the literature on the practical value of this are conflicting.[9,10,11]

Grading of cardiac rejection

There are numerous schemes for grading of cardiac rejection, many of which have contributed over the years to our overall understanding of the significance of particular pathological changes in biopsies of the post-transplant heart.[12] However, the following description will be confined to the ISHLT grading system[13] which has become widely adopted and, furthermore, most other grading systems can be readily translated into it (Table 7.4).

Adequacy of biopsies and technical considerations

A minimum of four endomyocardial biopsy fragments is stipulated with at least 50% of each free of biopsy site change or fibrosis. The role of fragment number in determining the "true" rejection grade has been established both on autopsy material and biopsy material.[14,15] From a clinical management point of view, however, it is often possible to give some useful information on less than four fragments. For instance, the features of significant rejection, i.e. 3A, 3B or 4, may be apparent on less than four fragments. On the other hand, when only three assessable fragments are present but all three are free of infiltrate the likelihood of missing significant underlying rejection is small and generally clinically acceptable.[15]

Tissue is formalin fixed and paraffin processed and sections are cut with a minimum recommendation of three levels through the block and three sections at each level stained with haematoxylin and eosin (H&E). A connective tissue stain may be performed at one of the levels and can be useful in identifying true fibrosis or myocyte damage, the latter being important in the early postoperative biopsies. However, a consistent quality of H&E staining is usually sufficient for adequate grading of the majority of biopsies. Most centres exceed the minimum requirements for sectioning. Serial sectioning with larger ribbons allows better assessment of small foci of cellular infiltration. An infiltrate that cuts out after a few serial sections is less significant than one that persists for many, this simply being a reflection of the volume of the infiltrate as well as its area in sections.

Grade 0 rejection

This grade is used for biopsies showing no infiltrate or only minimal scattered mononuclear infiltrates. Swollen endothelial cells and interstitial cell nuclei may be mistaken for infiltrating cells. However, as infiltrates of

Table 7.4   Grading of cardiac rejection ISHLT (1990)[13]

Old terms	Grade	Notes	Proposed simplification (1994)
No rejection	0	Biopsies with very sparse lymphoid infiltrates should be included in this grade	
"Mild" rejection	1A	Focal perivascular or interstitial infiltrates. The mild intensity and lack of myocyte damage distinguishes this from higher grades.	
	1B	Diffuse but sparse infiltrate. As with 1A, there must be no myocyte damage	Grade 1
"Focal" moderate rejection	2	One focus only with aggressive infiltration and/or focal myocyte damage. The choice of a single focus as the cut-off from higher grades is arbitrary. In practice, with the amount of tissue usually submitted, one is unlikely to be faced with the problem of biopsy fragments with only two foci	
		Usual treatment threshold	
"Low" moderate rejection	3A	Multifocal aggressive infiltrates and/or myocyte damage. The multiple foci may be present in only one fragment or may be scattered throughout several fragments	Grade 3A
	3B	Diffuse inflammatory process. The intensity of the lymphoid infiltrate varies considerably. It may be little more than 1B, the important feature distinguishing it being the presence of myocyte damage. This damage must be present in least two fragments, but some degree of infiltration is present in the majority of fragments	Grade 3B
"Severe acute" rejection	4	A diffuse and polymorphous infiltrate with or without oedema, haemorrhage, and vasculitis. The infiltrate is more intense and more widespread then 3B and myocyte damage is conspicuous. There are often neutrophils and/or haemorrhage, though neither is essential for diagnosis of this grade	Grade 4

this degree are clinically unimportant there is no need to resolve the issue by staining for leucocyte common antigen. Infiltrates may also be seen in intramyocardial or epicardial fat or scar and these should also be graded as 0.

Grade 1 rejection

Grade 1A and grade 1B rejection represent mild focal and diffuse mononuclear cell infiltrate respectively (Figures 7.1 and 7.2) Longitudinal studies have shown that these two histological patterns are not associated with different outcomes and consequently there is little point in distinguishing them.[16] In either case the mild nature of the infiltrate is characterised by its lack of intensity and failure to encroach on and, by inference, damage myocytes. The useful histological pointers in assessing these features are described below in relation to moderate grades of rejection.

Histological identification of moderate rejection

These criteria apply whether they relate to a single focus in a biopsy set, as in grade 2 rejection, or multiple foci as in grade 3A. Many previous grading systems have focused on the concept of recognising myocyte necrosis in order to diagnose moderate rejection. This has led to difficulties in the past, at least some of which may relate to the fact that the immune-mediated myocyte damage of rejection is more likely to be manifest as the

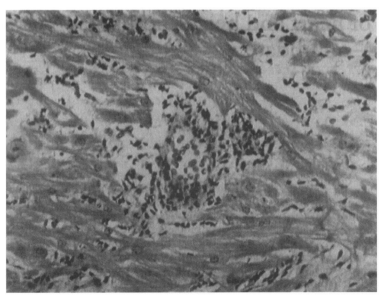

Fig 7.1   Grade 1A acute cardiac rejection: a focal mononuclear cell infiltrate, in this case perivascular. Haematoxylin and eosin (H&E).

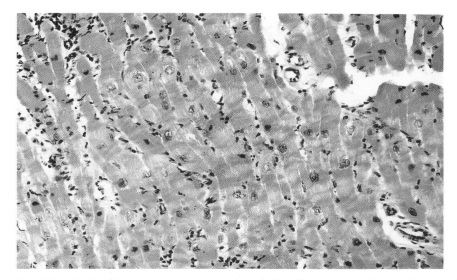

Fig 7.2   Grade 1B acute cardiac rejection: mild diffuse interstitial infiltrates (H&E).

less conspicuous process of apoptosis than necrosis. The ISHLT grading system requires an "aggressive" lymphoid infiltrate.[13] In practice, this is based on an assessment of both intensity of infiltrate and its relationship to myocytes. Intensity of infiltrate is seen both as area of myocardium involved in sections and persistence through several serial sections or even from one level to another. Myocyte damage is inferred from replacement of myocytes by infiltrate, with surrounding of individual myocytes and with mono-nuclear cells within myocyte cytoplasm (Figure 7.3). There is no specific need to see true myocyte *necrosis*. The infiltrate itself is mainly a mixture of T cells and macrophages. The relative proportions of CD4 versus CD8 T cells are variable, with both capable of participating in immune-mediated myocyte damage. Eosinophils may be present in small numbers in all grades of rejection, though they are more likely to accompany the infiltrate seen in 3A, 3B, and 4. Very occasional neutrophils may be seen in 3A and 3B though they are more likely to be present in grade 4.

Grade 2 rejection

This is defined as a single focus of moderate rejection throughout a whole biopsy set. The choice of one focus is clearly entirely arbitrary. The purpose of introducing this grade, however, was to define the histological entity where changes of moderate rejection were extremely focal and therefore unlikely to need treatment with enhanced immunosuppression. Experience

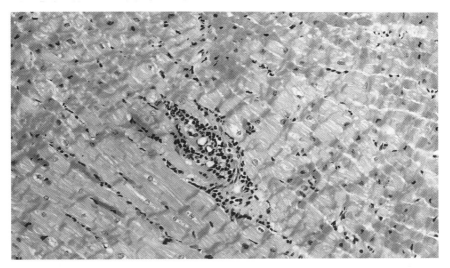

Fig 7.3   Grade 2 acute cardiac rejection: a focus of aggressive lymphoid infiltrate. Compared with figure 7.1, the infiltrate is encroaching on and by inference damaging a few myocytes (H & E).

has shown this to be the case and in a majority of biopsies the appearances of a single focus of moderate rejection may in fact be due to tangential cutting of encroaching endocardial infiltrates and therefore not rejection at all.[17] Such examples would not benefit from enhanced immunosuppression and any centre pitching the treatment threshold for rejection at grade 2 risks over immunosuppression. It has been our experience and that of others[18,19] that grade 2 rejection, whatever its true nature, is a benign entity that generally does not require enhanced immunosuppression.

Grade 3A rejection

This is defined as two or more foci of moderate rejection. The foci may be entirely confined to one fragment or may be spread through several fragments (Figure 7.4). The foci themselves must each independently fulfil the criteria for moderate rejection described above and this is clearly relevant in distinguishing this grade from grade 1A and grade 2. Compared to grade 3B, the background myocardium between foci should be clean and largely free of infiltrate. The main differential diagnosis to consider is opportunistic infection, in particular toxoplasmosis. In practice, however, this is rare nowadays as prophylaxis given to mismatched patients prevents significant toxoplasma myocarditis. Toxoplasma myocarditis compared to rejection tends to be a more mixed infiltrate, often including plasma cells and toxoplasma cysts (see later).

101

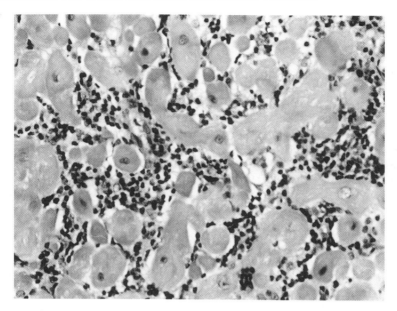

Fig 7.4   Grade 3A acute cardiac rejection: multiple foci of aggressive lymphoid infiltrates (H & E).

Grade 3B rejection

This is defined as a diffuse mononuclear cell infiltrate which should be seen in most or all of the biopsy fragments and associated with features of myocyte damage (as described under moderate rejection above) in at least two fragments. Compared to grade 3A rejection, the infiltrate may not be quite so intense and it is the diffuseness of the infiltrate and its association with myocyte damage that characterises this grade (Figure 7.5). Because of this the main differential diagnosis to consider in cases of 3B rejection is not 3A but rather 1B rejection. Difficulties may be encountered assessing this differential diagnosis early after transplantation when there may be scattered foci of myocyte damage related to peritransplant injury, in a background of diffuse mild rejection. Difficulty may also occur when some enhanced immunosuppression in the form of steroids has been given prior to biopsy, this having the effect of reducing the intensity of the diffuse cellular infiltrate. In view of these potential difficulties, when reporting such biopsies it is clearly important to have knowledge of the patient's clinical status, including time after transplant and whether or not enhanced immunosuppression has been given.

Apart from grade 1B rejection and peritransplant injury, there is little other differential diagnosis to consider in a process which is so widespread, affecting most or all of the biopsy fragments. Opportunistic infection generally tends to produce more focal infiltrates.

102

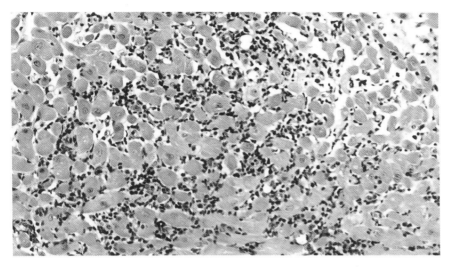

Fig 7.5 Grade 3B acute cardiac rejection: diffuse aggressive lymphoid infiltrate. The diffuse nature of the process distinguishes this from grade 3A and in a single field the process may seem similar (H & E).

Grade 4 rejection

There is a continuum from grade 3B to grade 4. Grade 4 simply represents a process which is more widespread, generally more intense, and is likely to include the presence of neutrophil polymorphs and haemorrhage though neither is essential to diagnose this grade. Infiltration is also often associated with destructive vasculitis. Cases of rejection at the borderline between 3B and 4 are occasionally seen, but florid grade 4 rejection is highly unlikely nowadays with modern immunosuppressive regimes. There are two important differential diagnoses to consider. Inflammatory granulation tissue and/or organising white thrombus-related previous biopsy sites may mimic the changes of grade 4 rejection and in order to make this diagnosis it is essential that the changes should be present in all fragments and that at least some of the fragments should be clearly independent of biopsy site changes. The other differential diagnosis to consider when coronary occlusive disease develops late on is myocardial infarction which is usually readily distinguishable due to the extent of myocardial necrosis compared to the degree of infiltration.

Resolving and resolved rejection

Resolving rejection is implied by the denoting of a lower grade of rejection in a follow-up biopsy following a treated rejection episode and similarly resolved rejection is denoted by grade 0 on follow-up biopsy.

However, there is no positive histological method of diagnosing resolving rejection.

Additional features seen on endomyocardial biopsy

Endocardial infiltrates

Endocardial infiltrates are common in the posttransplanted heart. They may be very mild and limited entirely to the endocardium (Figure 7.6) or they may be very florid and on occasion encroach on and damage underlying myocardium (Figure 7.7) as in the case of the Quilty lesions originally described by Billingham.[13] Perhaps surprisingly, even the most florid lesions appear to be associated with a benign outcome.[20] Furthermore, long-term studies have shown no difference between endocardial infiltrates which encroach on underlying myocardium (Quilty A) and those that do not (Quilty B).[20] Biopsies may be seen where infiltrate is entirely confined to the endocardium and subendocardial region with no evidence whatsoever of rejection in deeper myocardium. On the other hand, endocardial infiltrates may be seen in association with rejection of the deep myocardium and this should be graded in the normal way. Most higher grades of rejection, i.e. 3A, 3B or 4, are associated with significant endocardial infiltration.

In the more florid endocardial infiltrates there may be quite large dilated vessels with high endothelium and the lesion has the appearance of lymphoid tissue. Cellular composition is quite variable, plasma cells may be prominent and the lymphoid component may be quite pleomorphic.

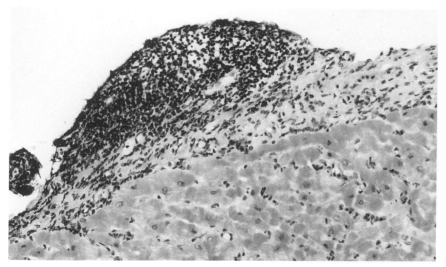

Fig 7.6 Endocardial lymphoid infiltrate, no encroachment on underlying myocardium (H & E).

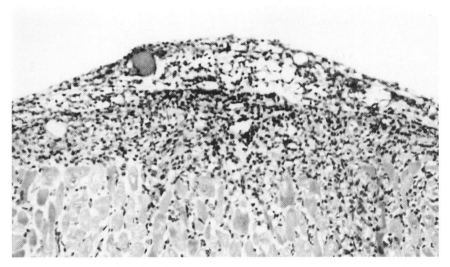

Fig 7.7 Endocardial lymphoid infiltrate with encroachment on underlying myocardium (H & E).

However, severe pleomorphism and/or atypia should always raise the possibility of infiltration of the endocardium by lymphoproliferative disease.[21]

Peritransplant injury

Early biopsies posttransplant often show small focal areas of myocyte damage, particularly in the subendocardial region. Initially there may be little if any cellular reacton, damage then resolves with the infiltration of macrophages. These lesions are best termed peritransplant injury as they may relate to endogenous catecholamines in the donor, e.g. in severe head injury or subarachnoid haemorrhage, or to exogenously administered catecholamines to either the donor or recipient posttransplant. Furthermore, reperfusion injury may produce similar small foci of myocyte damage. As foci of myocyte damage, they may cause difficulty in relation to the differential diagnosis of rejection as described above and knowledge of the time of transplantation is important. The differential diagnosis from rejection is made particularly difficult when such lesions resolve with a cellular infiltrate. In some individuals these areas heal by calcification. Some early posttransplant biopsies show concomitant acute rejection and peritransplant injury.

Infection

Compared to other solid-organ transplants, the likelihood of involvement of the transplanted heart by infection is remote. Opportunistic infection in

105

heart transplant recipients, however, often involves the lung and the pathology of these infections is covered later. CMV myocarditis appears to be rare even in those showing evidence in other organs of widely disseminated CMV disease.

Fungal infections may on occasion involve the heart in those with widely disseminated disease, usually as a consequence of heavy immunosuppression, and these may on rare occasions be biopsied. Some specific infections may, however, conspicuously involve the heart and toxoplasma myocarditis was an important cause of morbidity and mortality in the past in relation to those who were mismatched, that is, antibody-negative recipients of organs from antibody-positive donors.[22] Cardiac muscle represents a significant reservoir of infection in such donors with a high incidence of transmission compared to other solid-organ grafts and also a high mortality in such cases. However, knowledge of donor and recipient status, together with pyremethamine and more recently co-trimoxazole prophylaxis has eliminated this problem and cases are only likely to be seen if errors occur in relation to matching serology and prophylaxis. Myocardial involvement is common in primary toxoplasmosis[22] and, compared to rejection, the infiltrate appears to be more mixed. The associated toxoplasma cysts tend to be seen away from the areas of most intense inflammation and can easily be missed if the possibility of toxoplasmosis is not considered (Figure 7.8).

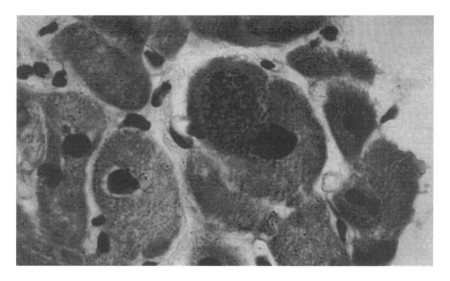

Fig 7.8   Toxoplasma cyst in routine follow-up endomyocardial biopsy specimen at seven years posttransplant. In other areas there were changes indistinguishable from grade 3A acute rejection, unlikely at this time after transplant. The patient had developed and recovered from primary toxoplasmosis postoperatively as a result of donor/recipient mismatching (H & E).

Recrudescent toxoplasma infection may be seen in relation to immunosuppression of those already seropositive. However, in practice infection is milder and not apparently associated with myocardial involvement.[22]

Clinical manifestations of rejection

Grades 3B and 4 are likely to be associated with cardiovascular symptoms and signs, particularly the latter which is usually associated with severe heart failure. Grade 3A may be accompanied by symptoms and signs of heart failure but is frequently seen in protocol biopsies in asymptomatic patients. The rationale in treating patients with asymptomatic 3A rejection is firstly to prevent potentially fatal dysrhythmia and secondly to prevent progression of rejection to a potentially irreversible stage with full-blown heart failure. Grades 1A, 1B and 2 are highly unlikely to produce cardiovascular symptoms or signs and when myocardial sampling is considered adequate, another cause must be sought.

Pathology and grading of acute pulmonary rejection

Grafted lungs have a high incidence of acute rejection when compared to other solid-organ allografts and this is most reliably diagnosed by transbronchial biopsy.[6,21,23,24,25] The Lung Rejection Study Group of the ISHLT has recommended that at least five pieces of alveolated lung parenchyma are examined to confidently grade acute pulmonary rejection.[25] In practical terms the bronchoscopist should submit more than five biopsies in order to provide this minimum number of parenchymal pieces. The biopsy fragments can be gently agitated in formalin to inflate them and may be processed according to a two-hour schedule if urgent. Sections from at least three levels of the paraffin block should be examined with H&E stains. This is, however, a minimum standard and many centres, including ours, examine multiple serial sections of the pulmonary biopsies. Connective tissue stains are essential for the diagnosis of airway and vascular fibrosis when chronic rejection is suspected and silver stains are mandatory for fungi and pneumocystis in all biopsies. Acute pulmonary rejection is manifest by perivascular infiltrates which increase in density and frequency with increasing severity.[6,21,25] A standardised nomenclature for its grading was established in 1990 by the Lung Rejection Study Group of the ISHLT (Table 7.5) and this was modified in 1995 in the light of experience of several large lung transplant centres (Table 7.6).[26] The diagnosis and grading of acute rejection are based exclusively on perivascular infiltrates.

Table 7.5 Working formulation for classification and grading of pulmonary rejection (1990)[25]

Grade A Acute rejection

A1	Minimal	
A2	Mild	
A3	Moderate	
A4	Severe	

Additional suffices
a With evidence of bronchiolar inflammation
b Without evidence of bronchiolar inflammation
c With large airway inflammation
d No bronchioles are present

Grade B Active airway damage without scarring
B) 1 Lymphocytic bronchitis   2 Lymphocytic bronchiolitis
       NO perivascular infiltrates, i.e. no A grade

Grade C Chronic airway damage with scarring
C) 1 Bronchiolitis obliterans– subtotal   2 Bronchiolitis obliterans–total
       a Active   a Active
       b Inactive   b Inactive
i.e. differs from B by having FIBROSIS

Grade D Chronic vascular rejection
Fibrointimal thickening of arteries and veins

Grade E Vasculitis
Necrosis of vessel wall disproportionate to other inflammation

---

Airway inflammation and its relationship to acute rejection are considered later.

Grade 0 rejection

This grade is used for biopsies free of mononuclear infiltrates or those showing such sparse infiltrates, which are not particularly perivascular, that they are not considered significant. Care must be taken not to overdiagnose bronchial mucosa-associated lymphoid tissue (BALT) as a pathological infiltrate, particularly on tangential cutting.

Table 7.6 Revised working formulation for classification and grading of lung allograft rejection[26]

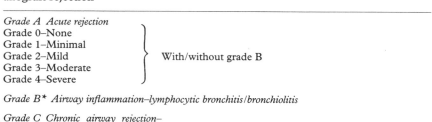

Grade A Acute rejection
Grade 0–None
Grade 1–Minimal
Grade 2–Mild   With/without grade B
Grade 3–Moderate
Grade 4–Severe

Grade B* Airway inflammation–lymphocytic bronchitis/bronchiolitis

Grade C Chronic airway rejection–
bronchiolitis obliterans
       a Active
       b Inactive

Grade D Chronic vascular rejection–accelerated graft vascular sclerosis

---

* Pathologist may choose to grade
B lesions B0–4, none–severe

Grade A1 rejection (minimal acute rejection)

This is the lowest grade of acute pulmonary rejection and is characterised by scattered infrequent perivascular mononuclear cell infiltrates which are not obvious at scanning magnification. Two to three cells in thickness infiltrate the perivascular adventitia and comprise small round and occasional plasmacytoid lymphocytes (Figure 7.9). These changes are more frequently seen around venules than arterioles.

Grade 2 (mild acute rejection)

In this grade the perivascular mononuclear infiltrates are more frequent and denser and are therefore readily recognisable at low magnification. They surround both venules and arterioles with small lymphocytes and larger activated lymphocytes including plasmacytoid lymphocytes, macrophages, and some eosinophils (Figure 7.10). Infiltration of the endothelium by these mononuclear cells causes hyperplasia in the endothelium and is known as endothelialitis in common with the similar process in other solid-organ grafts. The perivascular interstitium is expanded by the inflammatory infiltrate but the cells do not spill over into the adjacent alveolar septa or airspaces. A *solitary* perivascular mononuclear infiltrate of sufficient size and intensity to be recognised at low magnification and demonstrating these histological features is included in grade A2 rejection.

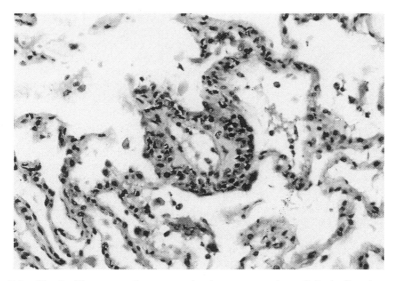

Fig 7.9 Grade A1 acute pulmonary rejection: scattered small foci of perivascular lymphoid infiltration. No lymphoid infiltration of bronchioles was present in these specimens, the complete grade therefore being A1, BO (H & E).

109

Grade A3 (moderate acute rejection)

In grade A3 the infiltrates are denser and generally more frequent and show conspicuous endothelialitis (Figure 7.11). Eosinophils and neutrophils are more common than in grade 2 and the defining feature is extension of the inflammatory infiltrate into perivascular alveolar septa and air spaces (Figure 7.12). Alveolar macrophages are commonly seen in the adjacent alveoli.

Grade A4 (severe acute rejection)

Grade A4 shows diffuse perivascular, interstitial and air space infiltrates of mononuclear cells with fewer small mature cells and proportionately more large activated lymphocytes. There is alveolar epithelial cell damage associated with hyaline membranes, haemorrhage, and conspicuous neutrophils (Figure 7.13). There may ultimately be parenchymal necrosis, infarction or a necrotising vasculitis.

Differential diagnosis of perivascular and interstitial infiltrates

Perivascular and interstitial mononuclear infiltrates are not histologically specific for acute rejection. Many other conditions may mimic acute pulmonary rejection and the important differential diagnoses to be

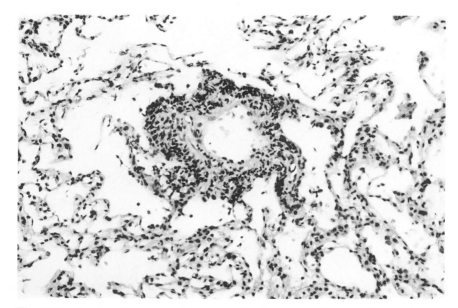

Fig 7.10 Grade A2 acute pulmonary rejection: more frequent larger foci of perivascular lymphoid infiltration (visible on scanning magnification) than grade A1 (H & E).

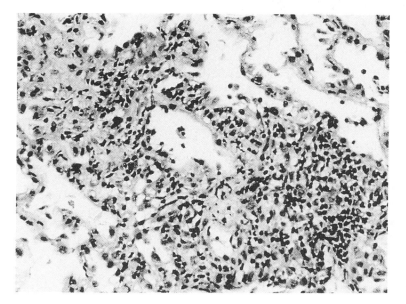

Fig 7.11   Grade A3 acute pulmonary rejection: changes of A2 with extension into surrounding interstitium. Endothelialitis is prominent (H & E).

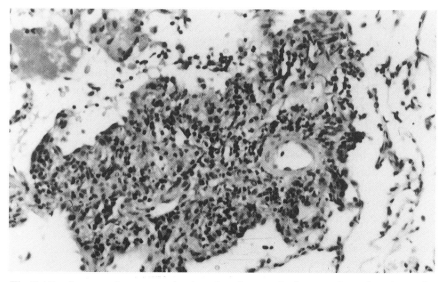

Fig 7.12   Acute pulmonary rejection showing marked expansion of perivascular adventitial tissue and early percolation of lymphoid cells into alveolar septa. There is an alveolar reaction with fibrin and mononuclear cells confirming that this is grade A3 rejection (H & E).

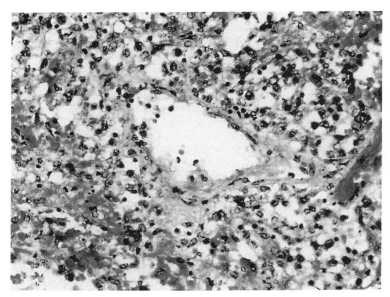

Fig 7.13 Grade A4 pulmonary rejection: extensive perivascular, interstitial and intraalveolar lymphoid infiltrates with intraalveolar fibrin. Polymorphs are also present together with some haemorrhage (H & E).

considered include opportunistic infection, particularly CMV and pneumocystis, posttransplant lymphoproliferative disease, which can range from pneumonitis to malignant lymphoma, bronchus-associated lymphoid tissue, and recurrent primary disease.[27] Endothelialitis is often a useful pointer to acute rejection as the cause of perivascular mononuclear infiltrate (Figure 7.14).

Acute pulmonary rejection involving airways

The basis for grading acute pulmonary rejection is the severity of the perivascular infiltrates in both the 1990 and 1995 schemes.[25,26] Accompanying the perivascular infiltrates there are often peribronchial and peribronchiolar infiltrates, the latter frequently seen on transbronchial biopsy material. Involvement of the airways is seen more frequently in the higher grades of rejection. The histological features range from simple non-infiltrative mononuclear cell cuffing of the airways to infiltration of the mucosa, ulceration and loss of epithelium and ultimately mucosal necrosis (Figures 7.15–18). In the 1990 classification coexistent airway inflammation was designated by four suffices to indicate the presence or absence of bronchial or bronchiolar infiltrates but not to reflect the intensity of the inflammatory process (Table 7.5). The potential is recognised for acute airways rejection to precede obliterative bronchiolitis, i.e chronic airways

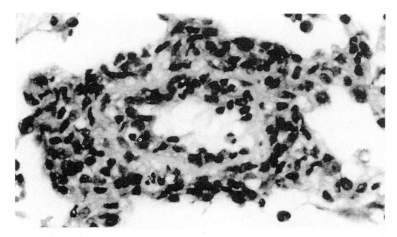

Fig 7.14 Grade A2 pulmonary rejection showing conspicuous endothelialitis which is rare in A1 (H & E). Endothelialitis is very uncommon in infection except in relation to endothelial CMV and then usually shows conspicuous admixed polymorphs (H & E).

rejection, and its importance is again emphasised in the 1995 classification.[26] Here airway inflammation is designated as category B which can be divided into five grades (0–4) according to intensity or simply designated as present or absent (Table 7.6). In practice, sampling problems and

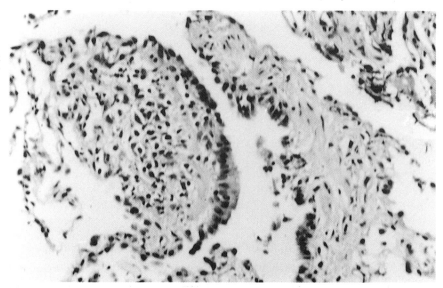

Fig 7.15 Lymphocytic bronchiolitis of minimal intensity. No perivascular infiltrates present nor evidence of infection. Grade AO, B1 (H & E).

113

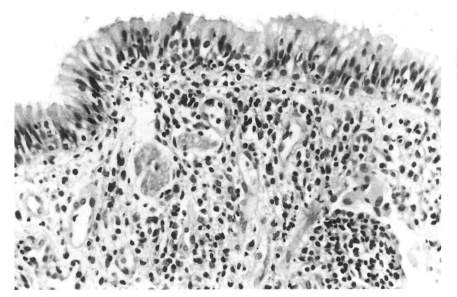

Fig 7.16 Lymphocytic bronchiolitis of mild intensity. Lymphocytes infiltrate epithelium but no epithelial damage is seen. Grade B2 (H & E).

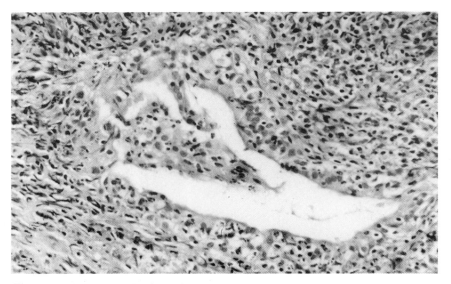

Fig 7.17 Lymphocytic bronchiolitis of moderate intensity with attenuated epithelium intact but including polymorphs and occasional eosinophils. Infection was excluded. Moderate perivascular infiltrates in the biopsy indicate grade A3, B3 (H&E).

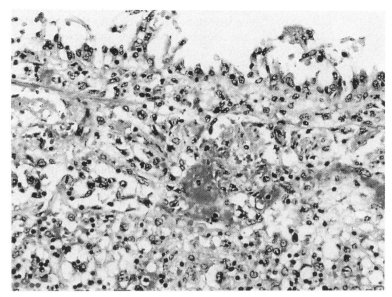

Fig 7.18 Severe lymphocytic bronchiolitis in a case of grade A4, B4 acute rejection showing destruction of epithelium by diffuse infiltrates (H & E).

tangential cutting together with the greater difficulty of excluding infection in the airways mean that many airway samples are ungradeable. These factors have also caused difficulties in establishing a link between acute airways rejection and obliterative bronchiolitis but it is agreed that, for grading purposes, its presence or absence should be documented in the absence of an infectious cause. For the purpose of everyday reporting of transbronchial biopsies, knowledge of the accompanying bronchial aspirate cytology is very helpful. A purulent aspirate with organisms demonstrated cytologically or by culture often helps interpretation of the biopsy airway inflammation as due to large airway infection. Grading bronchial/ bronchiolar samples in less than adequate biopsies should not be a substitute for assessing *adequate* parenchymal samples and assigning an A grade of acute rejection.

Concomitant acute pulmonary rejection and infection

There are several features of histological overlap between acute rejection and infection in the lung and in the case of *Pneumocystis carinii* pneumonitis the condition may be a close mimic of rejection.[28] Lung allografts have a high incidence of both common bacterial and opportunistic infections and these may occur concomitantly with acute rejection. The presence of an additional infective process effectively precludes grading and it is not possible to assign proportions of the inflammatory reaction to either

115

process. These biopsies should be reported as showing coexistent rejection and infection and it may be possible to favour one as the predominant process with experience.[29] These patients may require treatment with both augmented immunosuppression and appropriate antimicrobial therapy and there should be a low threshold for repeat biopsies if there is not an adequate response to treatment. There are, however, some histological features which are strongly in favour of an infective rather than a rejection process.

Granulomatous inflammation is not seen in pulmonary rejection and should immediately raise the possibility of opportunistic infection. The commonest organisms producing this type of reaction are pneumocystis, fungi exciting a bronchocentric granulomatous response, and mycobacteria. The liberal use of special stains and culture may be required to establish the correct diagnosis in the presence of such granulomatous inflammation. Only after meticulous exclusion of infection can the possibility of recurrence of sarcoidosis be considered in patients transplanted for that condition.[7,27]

Punctate areas of necrosis are also unusual in rejection and should again raise the possibility of infection, usually opportunistic and including particularly herpes simplex, aspergillus, and mycobacteria. Abundant neutrophils with the formation of microabscesses are a feature of cytomegalovirus pneumonitis in which perivascular oedema is generally more prominent than adventitial mononuclear cell infiltrates.[6,27]

Prominent infiltrates of eosinophils are also rare in acute rejection and should raise the possibility of infection, particularly by fungus.[30] The importance of close clinicopathological correlation cannot be over emphasised in lung transplantation pathology but it is critically important in the difficult area of distinguishing rejection from infection in patients requiring difficult therapeutic choices to be made.

Pathology of chronic rejection in the heart

Cardiomegaly is almost invariably seen in the long-term transplanted heart and repeated episodes of acute cellular rejection may result in interstitial fibrosis sufficient to affect cardiac function. However, the principal manifestation of chronic rejection is graft vascular disease and this remains the main factor limiting long-term survival of heart transplant recipients.[4] Compared to native atherosclerosis, graft vascular disease is more diffuse and progresses more rapidly. Involvement of secondary and tertiary epicardial coronary arteries is frequent. Nevertheless, involvement of the major epicardial arteries is important and rupture of atherosclerotic plaques in such vessels with resultant thrombosis appears to be a common terminal event in those dying of graft vascular disease.[4] It is likely that coronary graft disease is multifactorial. The disease in the larger epicardial arteries essentially resembles conventional atherosclerosis with lipid cores and macrophage foam cells and may well be an acceleration of preexisting donor atherosclerosis and preatherosclerosis. The disease involving the smaller epicardial coronary arteries, on the other hand, appears to be somewhat different in that lipid cores are not seen and vessels are obliterated partially or completely by intimal proliferation (Figure 7.19).

By its very nature coronary graft vascular disease only tends to be seen pathologically when it is endstage in patients either dying of it or being retransplanted for it. Consequently much of the pathological examination of occluded vessels provides little information about the factors precipitating and promoting occlusion. Nevertheless, in cases coming to retransplantation or in individuals dying of other causes who have some established coronary artery disease, it is possible to identify a proportion of coronary arteries with inflammatory infiltrates present in the intima associated with intimal proliferation. On this basis it is assumed that those vessels with endstage occlusion have gone through a similar inflammatory stage. The cellular infiltrates present in the intima of such vessels are a mixture of CD 4- and CD 8-positive T lymphocytes and it has been suggested that these may represent a chronic delayed hypersensitivity reaction associated with expression of HLA-DR by the T cells themselves and by the adjacent endothelium. This hypersensitivity reaction is proposed to result from CD 8-positive recipient T lymphocytes recognising class 1

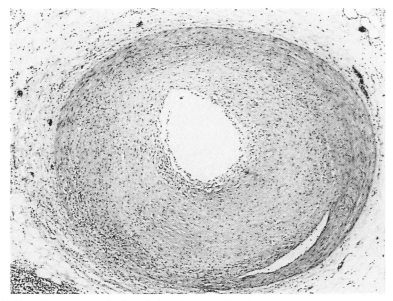

Fig 7.19 Coronary occlusive disease in a small epicardial artery showing cellular fibrointimal concentric proliferation (H&E).

expression by donor endothelium. The consequence of an intimal delayed hypersensitivity reaction would be the production of a variety of growth factors, leading to smooth muscle proliferation and secretion of extracellular material.

Indirect mechanisms involving the presentation of processed donor antigens by recipient cells may result in the production of a variety of antibodies and it has been suggested that such antibodies are a major factor in the pathogenesis of graft vascular disease. In relation to this possibility, HLA disparity between donor and recipient is inversely related to actuarial survival following transplant and, furthermore, those who develop anti-HLA antibodies have a much higher angiographic incidence of graft vascular disease.[31] The potential role of humoral mechanisms in acute graft malfunction has already been discussed and some have suggested that such humoral mechanisms are associated with subsequent development of graft vascular disease.[32-35] This may, however, at least in part, be explicable on the basis of sensitisation to mouse immunoglobulin due to the use of OKT3 antibody as a means of immunosuppression in those patients and unrelated to the underlying pathogenesis of graft vascular disease.[36]

As with acute rejection, it is likely that both cellular and humoral phenomena play a role in the development of coronary graft vascular disease. Endothelial and intimal damage by T cells may release antigens that subsequently give rise to an antibody response, which itself further accentuates damage.

Because endomyocardial biopsies generally do not sample epicardial coronary vessels there are few data examining the relationship between cellular infiltration of the intima of such vessels and cellular rejection of deep myocardium. Reports in the literature looking at the association between episodes of cellular rejection, i.e. myocardial rejection, and subsequent development of graft occlusive disease are conflicting.[37,38] However, even if cellular mechanisms are important in graft vascular disease, they cannot account entirely for the pathogenesis, as graft vascular disease has failed to decline despite considerable improvement in immunosuppressive regimes which are mainly aimed at acute cellular rejection. Whilst cellular and humoral immune mechanisms are likely to be the main underlying factors in the pathogenesis of graft vascular disease, there are other risk factors for development including peritransplant injury,[39] hyperlipidaemia,[40] and cytomegalovirus infection.[41]

Pathology of chronic pulmonary rejection

In common with other solid-organ grafts, the airways and vessels of the grafted lung can be involved in a fibroproliferative stenosing process with parenchymal fibrosis in the most advanced stages. The current major cause of long-term graft failure and death is chronic airways rejection where the pathological process involved is obliterative bronchiolitis (bronchiolitis obliterans).[2,42] Chronic vascular rejection of the lung assumes less clinical importance and shows histological features indistinguishable from those of coronary artery occlusive disease.

Obliterative bronchiolitis is a condition well recognised in non-transplanted lungs for which numerous causes have been described, many of which have a likely immunological basis.[43] When obliterative bronchiolitis occurs in the grafted lung it is considered to be the primary manifestation of chronic rejection, i.e. an immune process, but there are likely to be contributory factors including infection, ischaemia, denervation, and aspiration.[25,27,44] There is much evidence to support an immunological basis for obliterative bronchiolitis in the grafted lung in both animal and human studies. Clinically, repeated acute rejection episodes, acute airways rejection, persistent rejection, and high grades of acute rejection have all correlated with the development of obliterative bronchiolitis.[45,46,47] There is no consensus on the role of CMV infection, partly due to difficulties in distinguishing infection from disease in reports from various institutions, but there is no doubt that in the non-transplant population CMV can be associated with the development of obliterative bronchiolitis and it therefore remains a likely possibility.[47,48]

Class 2 antigens have been shown to be upregulated on the bronchiolar epithelium in lung transplant rejection and in patients with obliterative bronchiolitis.[49] Bronchoalveolar lavage has also demonstrated CD 8-positive non-cytotoxic cells directed against class 1 antigens.[50]

The diagnosis of obliterative bronchiolitis is often a combination of clinical and pathological features. The patients develop breathlessness and cough with a decline of their spirometry and this has been the basis of a classification of bronchiolitis obliterans syndrome (BOS) which can be graded according to severity.[51,54] On this clinical classification it is also noted whether or not there is histological confirmation of obliterative bronchiolitis on transbronchial biopsy material. Transbronchial biopsies are a relatively insensitive method of diagnosing obliterative bronchiolitis due to the patchy nature of the disease, particularly in its early stages, but the diagnostic yield can be enhanced by increasing the numbers of biopsies taken, the amount of tissue examined, and the liberal use of connective tissue stains to diagnose subtle changes of submucosal fibrosis which may otherwise be overlooked.[6,25,53,54,55] Transbronchial biopsies may be required in the later postoperative period to exclude other causes of pulmonary dysfunction including late acute rejection, opportunistic infection or lymphoproliferative disease, all of which can occur with OB. Infrequently, open-lung biopsy may be indicated in this setting with a yield of approximately 30% of new diagnoses that alter therapy.[56]

Obliterative bronchiolitis usually commences with fibrosis in the sub-epithelial region which expands the tissue between the epithelium and muscularis, firstly with granulation tissue and later with acellular fibrosis (Figure 7.20).[25] The overlying epithelium may be unchanged but more often becomes attenuated, metaplastic or ulcerated. The bronchiolar lumen may include granulation tissue. The stenosing luminal process is accompanied by fibroproliferative destruction of the bronchiolar muscle with fibrosis extending into the adventitia as either a patchy or diffuse process. The bronchiole may ultimately only be recognised by its proximity to an arteriole in elastic stained sections (Figure 7.21).[6,25,44] There may be distal mucostasis with foamy macrophages in air spaces but these foamy cells can also be seen as an integral part of the bronchiolar lesion. Rarely, obliterative bronchiolitis can develop within the first three months following transplantation but is not usually seen until the second postoperative year.

The 1990 Lung Rejection Study Group distinguished between subtotal and total forms of obliterative bronchiolitis as well as recording whether there was an accompanying active inflammatory infiltrate.[25] Experience with transbronchial biopsy material has shown, however, that sampling problems and tangential cutting cause difficulties in distinguishing subtotal and total forms and in the 1995 scheme bronchiolitis obliterans, grade C is described only as active or inactive according to any accompanying inflammatory infiltrate.[26] The obliterative process also involves cartilage-

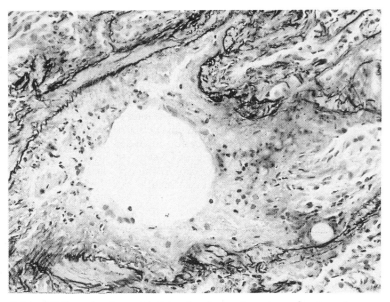

Fig 7.20 Obliterative bronchiolitis showing subtotal predominantly concentric narrowing by fibrous tissue including mononuclear inflammatory cells. Grade Ca (elastic van Gieson).

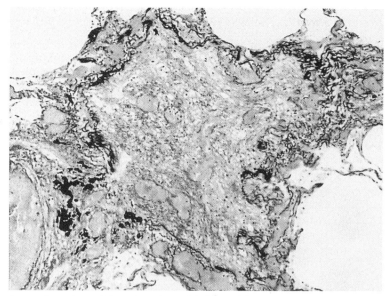

Fig 7.21 Inactive obliterative bronchiolitis with occluded lumen and intact bronchiolar elastica delineating airway structure (EVG).

containing airways and this may be seen on open biopsy or autopsy material but its functional significance is less certain.

Obliterative bronchiolitis due to chronic airways rejection should be distinguished from bronchiolitis obliterans organising pneumonia (BOOP) in which obliterative bronchiolitis is associated with intraluminal granulation tissue polyps and the involvement of distal parenchyma.[26,27] The two processes show little clinical or pathological overlap but it must be noted that lung transplant recipients can show organising pneumonia on transbronchial biopsy material due to infection or aspiration. This should not be confused with obliterative bronchiolitis. In difficult cases open biopsies may be required for assessment and it should be noted that patients can have OB and BOOP concomitantly.[58,59,60]

Chronic vascular rejection

Chronic vascular rejection in the lung consists of fibrointimal thickening of arteries and veins (Figure 7.22) with little clinical significance at the present time, obliterative bronchiolitis being the dominant pathological process. The graft vascular disease can be active or inactive and may correlate in combined heart-lung transplants with the presence of coronary artery occlusive disease.[25] Graft vascular disease within the lungs is often associated with obliterative bronchiolitis with which it shares a number of

121

pathological features. Pulmonary vascular disease may not be a manifestation purely of chronic rejection but could include reaction to preservation and ischaemic injury, parenchymal scarring, and thrombosis/embolism.

Pathology of opportunistic infection in heart and lung transplant patients

Heart and lung transplant recipients are very susceptible to opportunistic infection, particularly those with lung grafts. The recipients are also susceptible to common bacterial infections and the diagnosis and treatment of infections is a major management problem. Transbronchial biopsy has only a minor role in the diagnosis of bacterial infection although this may be suggested by a purulent inflammation in the airways or air spaces and the cytological features of the accompanying aspirate may point to the correct diagnosis whilst culture results are awaited. Transbronchial biopsy and lavage cytology are important in the diagnosis of opportunistic infections, particularly those due to virus and fungus.[6,24,51]

Cytomegalovirus

Cytomegalovirus (CMV) may be transmitted to the recipient in the graft or in blood or blood products as a primary infection. The virus may also be

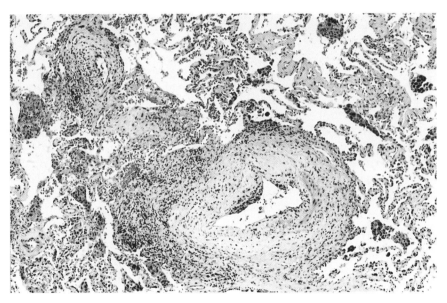

Fig 7.22 Pulmonary vascular occlusive disease of chronic rejection involving arterial branch. Fibroproliferative thickening is accompanied by transmural inflammation and endothelialitis. Venous involvement (not shown) is usually hyaline acellular sclerosis (EVG).

reactivated in a seropositive recipient to cause disease.[62] CMV pneumonitis as part of a generalised CMV infection is the most serious complication seen in lung and, to a lesser extent, heart recipients.[63] The classic appearances of CMV pneumonitis on transbronchial biopsy are those of viral alveolitis with diffuse alveolar damage in many cases. (Figure 7.23).[6,27] The prominent features are polymorphs in the interstitial infiltrate often congregating to form microabscesses. There are marked changes in the alveolar epithelial cells with reactive appearances and/or ulceration. Mononuclear cell infiltrates are not a feature and the vessels tend to show perivascular oedema. Diagnostic intranuclear "owl's eye" and granular intracytoplasmic inclusions allow a confident diagnosis to be made. The viral inclusions involve both alveolar epithelial and endothelial cells as well as alveolar macrophages. If the biopsy is taken prior to the development of diagnostic inclusions the features of viral alveolitis in the appropriate clinical setting can allow the diagnosis to be suggested.[6]

In the management of lung recipients prior to antiviral prophylaxis the diagnosis of CMV pneumonitis was usually straightforward. In the early days of transplant programmes CMV-positive organs transplanted into CMV-negative recipients often resulted in a fulminant CMV pneumonitis with systemic spread. The widespread use of prophylaxis with ganciclovir

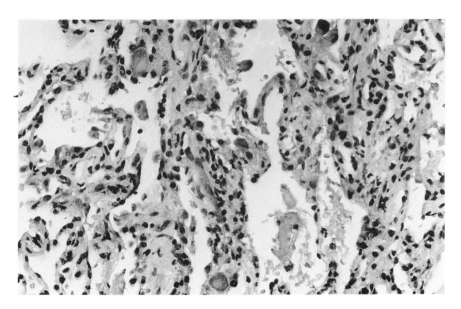

Fig 7.23 CMV pneumonitis with numerous enlarged cells showing intranuclear and faint intracytoplasmic inclusions. The viral alveolitis shows frequent polymorphs in the infiltrate and intraalveolar fibrin. The diffuseness and nature of the infiltrate distiguishes it from acute rejection (H & E).

has, however, modified the biopsy appearances. The commonest appearance now tends to be focal neutrophilic pneumonitis in which inclusions may not be obvious unless multiple serial sections are examined. The inclusions that develop in the presence of prophylactic antiviral therapy may not be readily recognisable in H&E stained sections. The infected cells may not show the characteristic gross enlargement and the intranuclear inclusions may be uncharacteristically eosinophilic and degenerate. Immunohistochemical staining for CMV may be helpful. Obviously good clinicopathological correlation is required under these circumstances to make the correct diagnosis.

The main differential diagnosis is from herpes simplex infection which is bronchopneumonic in distribution with necrosis and lack of cytomegaly and shows intranuclear inclusions only.[64] The distinction between CMV and herpes simplex in a problematic biopsy is another area where immunohistochemistry or *in situ* hybridisation may resolve a diagnostic dilemma.[65] However, the routine use of more sensitive specialised techniques for the diagnosis of CMV pneumonitis has not shown widespread benefits. Often, the inclusions which are easily recognised on H&E staining are confirmed without evidence of widespread latent infection. In the absence of an inflammatory infiltrate the presence of CMV inclusions in a seropositive recipient is of doubtful pathological significance and therefore methods that increase sensitivity of detection are not uniformly beneficial.[66,67] The presence of CMV inclusions in a bronchoalveolar lavage sample without evidence of virus or inflammation in the accompanying transbronchial biopsies is also insufficient for a diagnosis of CMV pneumonitis. It must be remembered that some patients will have systemic CMV disease with minimal pulmonary involvement and the absence of pulmonary disease should not preclude antiviral treatment. In lung transplant patients where CMV pneumonitis or infection exists with perivascular mononuclear infiltrates, a diagnosis of concomitant rejection/infection can be made but ISHLT grading is not possible.[25,26] Careful modulation of both antiviral and immunosuppressive therapy may be necessary with a low threshold for follow-up biopsy.

Pneumocystis carinii

The use of prophylactic regimes has similarly decreased the incidence of *Pneumocystis carinii* in cardiac and pulmonary transplant programmes. The diagnosis of pneumocystis in this group of patients can be problematic as the characteristic abundant intraalveolar foamy exudate seen in other groups of immunocompromised patients is not a prominent feature.[27] This group of patients tends to produce an atypical histological reaction, commonly granulomatous with a reduced number of organisms. The main histological finding can also be a mononuclear interstitial infiltrate closely mimicking acute rejection [28] hence the mandatory use of silver staining in biopsy material from lung transplant patients.[25] Other atypical reactions include acute lung injury of diffuse alveolar damage pattern.[68] Patients who are intolerant of prophylaxis or do not comply with therapy may develop clinically unsuspected *Pneumocystis carinii* and this important opportunistic pathogen which is readily treatable should not be overlooked.

Mycobacterial infection

Perhaps surprisingly, mycobacterial disease is not common in lung transplant recipients. Sporadic reports have appeared in the literature of both tuberculous and non-tuberculous mycobacterial disease.[6,69,70] However with the increasing survival of many patients and the wider range of conditions treated by transplantation, the incidence of mycobacterial disease appears to be increasing.

The histological features are generally those of granulomatous inflammation with or without necrosis and multiple sections should be examined with Ziehl–Neelsen and modified Ziehl–Neelsen stains as well as for culture. Occasionally necrosis without granulomas and showing prominent polymorphs is seen, this pattern having been recently identified at our hospital in a patient with multiple nodules due to *Mycobacterium kansasii* . The other atypical organisms encountered in our programme include *M. fortuitum, chelonae* and *malmaoense*. Patients with sarcoidosis may have recurrence of granulomas in transbronchial biopsy material but these should not be ascribed to recurrent primary disease until opportunistic infection, including mycobacterial infection, has been meticulously excluded.[6,7] One patient in our programme with sarcoidosis developed necrotising granulomas from which *Mycobacterium tuberculosis* was cultured, having had no previous evidence of tuberculosis, and this patient serves as a reminder of the complex relationship between sarcoidosis and tuberculosis. Patients with tuberculosis in explanted lungs, particularly single-lung recipients with a remaining native lung, may require anti-tuberculous chemotherapy to reduce the risk of tuberculosis developing posttransplantation.[5]

Aspergillus

Infection by aspergillus is a major clinical problem in most lung transplant programmes. The fungus is ubiquitous and causes a spectrum of diseases in this population ranging from colonisation to destructive invasive and widely disseminating disease.[71] For this reason, identification of fungus either by culture or microscopic examination of sputum or lavage fluid is inadequate to correctly define an individual's disease on this spectrum. It is important not to overtreat colonisation in view of the side effects of the antifungal treatment and the risk of the development of resistant strains.

Transbronchial biopsy material may demonstrate abundant eosinophils in those patients with an allergic bronchopulmonary aspergillosis or mucoid impaction with eosinophilic pneumonia.[30,71] Another histological pattern identified on biopsy is bronchocentric granulomatous mycosis in which multiple sections may have to be examined to identify the infrequent and often fragmented fungal hyphae.[73] Cavitation with necrosis and invasive aspergillus is relatively uncommon but indicates severe disease with marked potential for dissemination (Figure 7.24). Another life-threatening form is necrotising aspergillus pneumonia. Connective tissue stains are particularly useful in identifying vascular invasion for which this fungus has a particular propensity. In the postoperative period, any slough or degenerate cartilage in mucosal biopsies should be carefully scrutinised for evidence of aspergillus as invasion of ischaemic airways can be catastrophic with erosion of the pulmonary artery or dissemination.[73]

Lymphoproliferative disease

Posttransplant lymphoproliferative disease (LPD) is most often of B-cell type and related to Epstein–Barr virus (EBV) infection.[74] It is a well-recognised long-term complication of all solid-organ transplants and is frequent following heart and lung transplantation, particularly the latter.[75,76] This reflects the higher levels of immunosuppression required in this

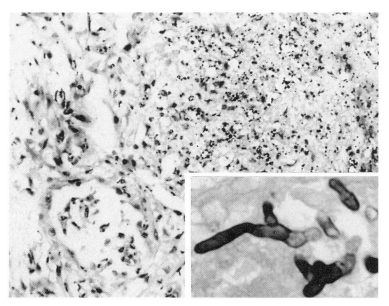

Fig 7.24 Invasive aspergillosis in the lung characterised by foci of necrosis in which hyphae are identifiable (H & E with Grocott methenamine silver, inset).

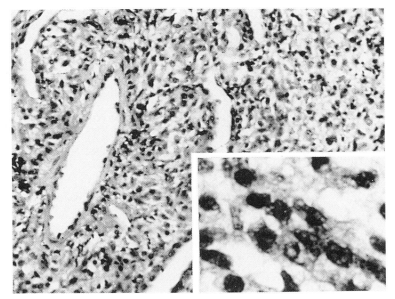

Fig 7.25 Lymphoproliferative disease in heart-lung transplant recipient diagnosed on transbronchial biopsy by sheet-like infiltrate of mixed lymphoid population showing cellular atypia, mitoses, and coagulative necrosis (features not seen in acute pulmonary rejection) (H & E).

group of patients. Extranodal involvement is common and, in heart recipients, may occur in the heart itself, often endocardially where it must be distinguished from benign endocardial infiltrates. In lung transplant recipients disease in the grafted organ itself is common and may present relatively soon after transplantation.[75] The patients may have non-specific or pulmonary symptoms with accompanying nodules on the chest X-ray and CT. Diagnosis by needle aspiration is difficult and cutting needle or transbronchial biopsies may be preferred in the first instance.[77]

Histologically, the infiltrate is more diffuse than that of acute pulmonary rejection with larger activated cells and coagulative necrosis (Figure 7.25).[75,76,78,79] In this setting the presence of coagulative necrosis is strongly suspicious of lymphoproliferative disease even if little viable material is present. The invasion of vessels with fibrinoid necrosis is also a distinguishing feature from acute pulmonary rejection. Morphologically B-cell lymphoproliferative disease may be of pleomorphic or monomorphic type.[80] Histologically aggressive-looking lymphoproliferation may nevertheless regress with a reduction in immunosuppression. However, cytotoxic chemotherapy and/or radiotherapy may be required.

127

References

1 Schofield PM. Indications for cardiac transplantation. *Br Heart J* 1991;**65**:55–6.

2 Hosenpud JD, Novick RJ, Bennett LE *et al.* The Registry of the International Society for Heart and Lung Transplantation: thirteenth official report *J Heart Lung Transplant* 1996;**15**:655–74.

3 Silver MA, Winters GL, Costanzo-Nordin MR *et al.* Eosinophilic myocarditis in heart transplant recipient hearts. *J Am Coll Cardiol* 1987;**9**:144A.

4 Mullins PA, Cary NR, Sharples L *et al.* Coronary occlusive disease in late graft failue after cardiac transplantation. *Br Heart J* 1992;**68**:260–5.

5 Stewart S, McNeil K, Nashef S *et al.* Audit of referral and explant diagnoses in lung transplantation: A pathological study of lungs removed for parenchymal disease. *J Heart Lung Transplant* 1995;**14**:1173–86.

6 Higenbottam TW, Stewart S, Penketh AR *et al.* Transbronchial lung biopsy for the diagnosis of rejection in heart-lung transplant patients. *Transplantation* 1988;**46**:532–9.

7 Johnson BA, Duncan SR, Ohori NO *et al.*, Recurrence of sarcoidosis in pulmonary allograft recipients. *Am Rev Respir Dis* 1993;**148**:1373–7.

8 Caves PK, Stinson EB, Billingham ME, Shumway NE. Percutaneous transvenous endomyocardial biopsy in human heart recipients (experience with a new technique). *Ann Thorac Surg* 1973;**16**:325.

9 Hammond ME, Yowell RL, Nuroda S *et al.* Vascular (humoral) rejection in heart transplantation: Pathologic observations and clinical implications. *J Heart Transplant* 1989;**8**:430–43.

10 Bonnaud EV, Lewis NP, Masek MA, Billingham ME. Reliability and usefulness of immunoflourescence in heart transplantation. *J Heart Lung Transplant* 1995;**14**:163–71.

11 Lones MA, Czer LSC, Trento A *et al.* Clinical-pathology features of humoral rejection in cardiac allografts: a study in 81 consecutive patients. *J Heart Lung Transplant* 1995;**14**:162–71.

12 Billingham ME. The dilemma of variety of histopathological grading systems for acute cardiac allograft rejection by endomyocardial biopsy. *J Heart Transplant* 1989;**9**:272–6.

13 Billingham ME, Cary NRB, Hammond ME *et al.* A working formulation for the standardization of nomenclature in the diagnosis of cardiac and lung rejection. *J Heart Transplant* 1990;**9**:587–93.

14 Zerbe T, Uretsky B, Kormos R *et al.* Graft atherosclerosis: effect of cellular rejection and human lymphocyte antigen. *J Heart Lung Transplant* 1992;**11**:S104-10

15 Sharples LD, Cary NRB, Large SR, Wallwork J. Error rates with which endomyocardial biopsies are graded for rejection following cardiac transplantation. *Am J Cardiol* 1992;**70**:527–30.

16 Riseq MN, Masek MA, Billingham ME. Acute rejection: significance of lapsed time post transplant. *J Heart Lung Transplant* 1994;**13**:862–8.

17 Fishbein MC, Bell G, Lones MA, *et al.* Grade 2 cellular rejection: does it exist? *J Heart Lung Transplant* 1994;**13**;1051–7.

18 Winters G, Loh E, Schoen F. Natural history of focal moderate cardiac allograft rejection. Is treatment warranted? *Circulation* 1995;**91**:1975–80.

19 Forbes RD, Rowan RA, Billingham ME. Endocardial infiltrates in human heart transplants: a serial biopsy analysis comparing full immunosuppression protocols. *Human Pathol* 1990;**21**:850–5.

20 Joshi A, Masek MA, Brown BW, Weiss LM, Billingham ME. Quilty revisited: a 10 year prospective. *Human Pathol* 1994;**26**:547–57.

21 Stewart S, Cary NRB. The pathology of heart and lung transplantation. *Curr Diagnost Pathol* 1996;**3**:69–79.

22 Wreghitt TG, Hackim M, Gray JJ *et al.* Toxoplasmosis in heart and heart-lung transplant recipients. *J Clin Pathol* 1989;**42**:194–9.

23 Hutter JA, Stewart S, Higenbottam TW *et al.* The characteristic histological changes associated with rejection in heart-lung transplant recipients. *Transplant Proc* 1989;**21**:435–6.

24 Guilinger RA, Paradis IL, Dauber JH *et al.* The importance of bronchoscopy with transbronchial biopsy and bronchoalveolar lavage in the management of lung transplant recipients. *Am J Respir Crit Care Med* 1995;**152**:2037–43.

25 Yousem SA, Berry GJ, Brunt EM *et al*. A working formulation for the standardization of nomenclature in the diagnosis of heart and lung rejection: Lung Rejection Study Group. *J Heart Transplant* 1990;**9**:593–601.

26 Yousem SA, Berry GJ, Cagle PT *et al*. A revision of the 1990 working formulation for the classification of lung allograft rejection. *J Heart Lung Transplant* 1996;**15**:1–15.

27 Stewart S. The pathology of lung transplantation. *Seminar Diagnost Pathol* 1992;**9**:210–19.

28 Tazelaar HD. Perivascular inflammation in pulmonary infections: implications for the diagnosis of lung rejection. *J Heart Lung Transplant* 1991;**10**:437–41.

29 Hunt JB, Stewart S, Cary NRB *et al*. Evaluation of the International Society for Heart Transplantation (ISHT) grading of pulmonary rejection in 100 consecutive biopsies. *Transplant Int* 1992;**1**:S249–S251.

30 Yousem SA. Graft eosinophilia in lung transplantation. *Human Pathol* 1992;**23**:1172–7.

31 Petrossian GA, Nichols AB, Marboe CC *et al*. Relation between survival and development of coronary artery disease and anti-HLA antibodies after cardiac transplantation. *Circulation* 1989;**80**(suppl):111–22.

32 Hammond EH, Ensley RD, Yowell RL *et al*. Vascular rejection of human cardiac allografts and the role of humoral immunity in chronic allograft rejection. *Transplant Proc* 1991;**23**:26.

33 Hess ML, Hastillo A, Mohanakumar T. Accelerated atherosclerosis in cardiac transplantation: Role of cytotoxic B-cell antibodies and hyperlipidaemia. *Circulation* 1983;**68**:Suppl II;94–101.

34 Ensley RD, Hammond EH, Renlund DG *et al*. Clinical manifestations of vascular rejection in cardiac transplantation. *Transplant Proc* 1991;**23**:1130–32.

35 Lones MA, Czerl SC, Tranter A *et al*. Clinical pathology features of humoral rejection in cardiac allograft: a study of 81 consecutive patients. *J Heart Lung Transplant* 1995;**14**:162–71.

36 Hammond EH, Yowell RL, Price GD *et al*. Vascular rejection and its relationship to allograft coronary artery disease. *J Heart Lung Transplant* 1992;**11**:S111–19.

37 Zerbe T, Uretsky B, Kormos R *et al*. Graft atherosclerosis: effect of cellular rejection and human lymphocyte antigen. *J Heart Lung Transplant* 1992;**11**:S104–10.

38 Gao SZ, Schroeder JS, Aderman ET *et al*. Prevalence of accelerated coronary artery disease in heart transplant survivors: comparison of cyclosporine and azathioprine regimens. *Circulation* 1989;**80**:III–100.

39 Gsaudin PB, Rayburn BK, Hutchins GM. Peritransplant injury to the myocardium associated with the development of accelerated arteriosclerosis in heart transplant recipients. *Am J Surg Pathol* 1994;**18**:338–46.

40 Parameshwar J, Foote J, Sharples L *et al*. Lipids, lipoprotein (a) and coronary artery disease in patients following cardiac transplant. *Transplant Int* 1996;**9**:481–5.

41 Everett JP, Hershberger RE, Norman DJ *et al*. Prolonged cytomegalovirus infection with viraemia is associated with development of cardiac allograft vasculopathy. *J Heart Lung Transplant* 1992;**11**:S133–7.

42 Burke CM, Theodore J, Dawkins KD *et al*. Post transplant obliterative bronchiolitis and other late lung sequelae in human heart-lung transplantation. *Chest* 1984;**86**:824–9.

43 Epler GR, Colby TV. The spectrum of bronchiolitis obliterans. *Chest* 1983;**83**:161–2.

44 Tazelaar HD, Yousem SA. The pathology of combined heart-lung transplantation. An autopsy study. *Human Pathol* 1988;**119**:1403–16.

45 Yousem SA, Dauber JA, Keenan R *et al*. Does histologic acute rejection in lung allografts predict the development of bronchiolitis obliterans? *Transplantation* 1991;**52**:306–9.

46 Scott JP, Higenbottam TW, Sharples L *et al*. Risk factors of obliterative bronchiolitis in heart-lung transplant recipients. *Transplantation* 1991;**51**:813–17.

47 Sharples L, Scott J, Dennis C *et al*. Risk factors for survival following combined heart-lung transplantation. *Transplantation* 1994;**57**:218–23.

48 Colby TV. Bronchiolar pathology. In: Epler GR. ed. *Diseases of the Bronchioles* New York: Raven Press, 1994.

49 Burke CM, Glanville AR, Theodore J *et al*. Lung immunogencity, rejection and obliterative bronchiolitis. *Chest* 1987;**92**:547–9.

129

50 Reinsmoen NL, Bolman RM, Savile K *et al.* Differentiation of class I and class II-directed donor-specific alloreactivity in bronchoalveolar lavage lymphocytes from lung transplant recipients. *Transplantation* 1992;**53**:181–9.

51 Cooper JD, Billingham M, Egan T *et al.* A working formulation for the standardization of nomenclature and for clinical staging of chronic dysfunction in lung allografts. *J Heart Lung Transplant* 1993;**12**:713–16.

52 Keller CA, Cagle PT, Brown RW, Noon G, Frost AE. Bronchiolitis obliterans in recipients of single, double and heart-lung transplantation. *Chest* 1995;**107**:973–80.

53 Yousem SA, Paradis I, Griffith BP. Can transbronchial biopsy aid in the diagnosis of bronchiolitis obliterans in lung transplant recipients? *Transplantation* 1994;**57**:151–3.

54 Cagle PT, Brown RW, Frost A, Kellar C, Yousem SA. Diagnosis of chronic lung transplant rejection by transbronchial biopsy. *Modern Pathol* 8.2:137–42.

55 Reichenspurner H, Girgis RE, Robbins RC *et al. Ann Thorac Surg* 1996;**62**:1467–73.

56 Chaparro C, Maurer JR, Chamberlain DW, Todd TR. Role of open lung biopsy for diagnosis in lung transplant recipients: ten-year experience. *Ann Thorac Surg* 1995;**59**:928–32.

57 Yousem SA, Duncan S, Griffith B. Interstitial and airspace granulation tissue reaction in lung transplant recipients. *Am J Surg Pathol* 1992;**16**:877–84.

58 Milne DS, Gascoigne AD, Ashcroft T *et al.* Organising pneumonia following pulmonary transplantation and the development of obliterative bronchiolitis. *Transplantation* 1994;**57**:1757–62.

59 Chaparro C, Chamberlain D, Maurer J *et al.* Bronchiolitis obliterans organising pneumonia (BOOP) in lung transplant patients. *Chest* 1996;**110**:1150–4.

60 Siddiqui MT, Garrity ER, Husain AN. Bronchiolitis obliterans organising pneumonia-like reactions: a non-specific response or an atypical form of rejection or infection in lung allograft recipients. *Human Pathol* 1996;**27**:714–19.

61 Chan CC, Abi-Saleh WJ, Arroliga AC *et al.* Diagnostic yield and therapeutic impact of flexible bronchoscopy in lung transplant recipients. *J Heart Lung Transplant* 1996;**15**:196–205.

62 Smyth RL, Scott JP, Borysiewicz LK *et al.* Cytomegalovirus infection in heart-lung transplant recipients: risk factors, clinical associations and response to treatment. *J Infect Dis* 1991;**164**:1045–50.

63 Wreghitt TG, Hakim M, Gray JJ, Kucia S, Wallwork J. Cytomegalovirus infections in heart and heart and lung transplant recipients. *J Clin Pathol* 1988;**41**:660–7.

64 Smyth RL, Higenbottam TW, Scott JP *et al.* Herpes simplex virus infection in heart-lung transplant recipients. *Transplantation* 1990;**49**:735–9.

65 Weiss LM, Movahed LA, Berry GJ *et al.* In situ hybridization studies for viral nucleic acids in heart and lung allograft biopsies. *Am J Clin Pathol* 1990;**93**:675–9.

66 Myerson D, Hackman RC, Nelson JA *et al.* Widespread presence of histologically occult cytomegalovirus. *Human Pathol* 1984;**15**:430–9.

67 Niedobiteck G, Finn T, Herbst H *et al.* Detection of cytomegalovirus by in-situ hybridisation and histochemistry using a monoclonal antibody CCH2: 1 comparison of methods. *J Clin Pathol* 1988;**41**:1005–9.

68 Weber WR, Askin FB, Dehner LP. Lung biopsy in pneumocystis carinii pneumonia. A histological study of typical and atypical features. *Am J Clin Pathol* 1977;**67**:11–19.

69 Dromer C, Nashef SAM, Velly J-F, Matigne C, Couraud L. Tuberculosis in transplanted lungs. *J Heart Lung Transplant* 1993;**12**:924–7.

70 Trulock EP, Bolman RM, Genton R. Pulmonary disease caused by mycobacterium chelonae in a heart-lung transplant recipient with obliterative bronchiolitis. *Am Rev Respir Dis* 1989;**140**:802–5.

71 S Stewart. Pathology of lung transplantation. In: Sheppard MN. ed. *Practical pulmonary pathology*. London: Edward Arnold, 1995.

72 Tazelaar HD, Baird AM, Mill M *et al.* Bronchocentric mycosis occurring in transplant recipients. *Chest* 1989;**96**:92–5

73 Kramer MR, Denning DW, Marhall SE *et al.* Ulcerative tracheobronchitis after lung transplantation. *Am Rev Respir Dis* 1991;**144**:552–6.

74 Penn I. Cancers complicating organ transplantation. *N Engl J Med* 1990;**323**:1767–8.

75 Coueteil JP, McGoldrick JP, Wallwork J, English TAH. Malignant tumours after heart transplantation. *J Heart Transplant* 1990;**9**:622–6.

76 Yousem SA, Randhawa P, Lock J *et al*. Posttransplant lymphoproliferative disorders in heart-lung transplant recipients. *Human Pathol* 1989;**20**:361–9.

77 End A, Helbich T, Wisser W, Dekan G, Kleptoko W. The pulmonary nodule after lung transplantation. Cause and outcome. *Chest* 1995;**107**:117–22.

78 Rosendale B, Yousem SA. Discrimination of Epstein-Barr virus-related post transplant lymphoproliferations from acute rejection in lung allograft recipients. *Arch Pathol Lab Med* 1995;**119**:418–23.

79 Randhawa PS, Yousem SA. Epstein-Barr virus-associated lymphoproliferative disease in a heart-lung allograft. *Transplantation* 1990;**49**:126–30.

80 Nalesnik MA. Post transplantation lymphoproliferative disorders (PTLD): current perspectives. *Semin Thorac Cardiovasc Surg* 1996;**8**:139–48.

131

8 General management of the heart transplant recipient

Jayan Parameshwar

Heart transplantation has evolved from an experimental procedure to an established treatment for patients with severe heart failure refractory to medical management. When recipients and donors are carefully selected operative mortality is now less than 5% in well-established transplant units and one-year survival is 90%.[1] To maximise long-term survival and minimise complications of immunosuppressive therapy, it is important to organise the long-term management of the patients carefully. More than for any other surgical procedure, there needs to be a commitment to meticulous lifelong follow-up by the transplant team.

The transplant continuing care unit

At Papworth Hospital, a transplant continuing care unit was set up nearly 10 years ago. The transplant physician or cardiologist is ideally involved in the selection of patients for transplantation along with the nursing staff in the unit who are likely to provide a large proportion of the long-term care required. Perhaps more than in other areas of medicine, continuity of care is important to enable problems to be identified and dealt with as early as possible. Such continuity also engenders confidence in the patient and in the primary care physicians and referring physicians involved in patient care. Ensuring prompt and detailed communication with other health-care workers is extremely important in this regard. Patients are encouraged to contact us however minor their symtoms may be. A nurse on the continuing care unit deals with the problem on the telephone when possible; when appropriate, the patient is advised to contact the general practitioner. A physician who knows the patient is usually available in the unit to deal with questions if required. Finally, any patient who requests an early visit to the unit is always accommodated.

Intermediate care

At Papworth Hospital, patients are usually discharged from the ward to an "intermediate care" area. In our case this consists of a house in the local village about 600 m from the hospital. The house accommodates up to four couples; patients stay there for 3–7 days with their partner and are seen in the continuing care unit every other day or as required. Patients (and their partners) find this system invaluable in building up their confidence before going home. The intermediate care area is particularly useful for patients who live relatively far away for whom frequent visits to hospital are impractical.

Patient Education

At Papworth we believe the education of the patient starts at the assessment admission. Patients are told in great detail about the problems they may experience both early and late after cardiac transplantation. After the transplant the nursing staff in the continuing care unit have the responsibility of ensuring that the patients understand the reason for each of their drugs and the possible side effects. They are also instructed in the possible symptoms of acute rejection and infection so that they can call for help early. Patients maintain a diary which lists their medication, weight, blood pressure, and any symptoms they experience. We have found this invaluable in confirming that patients have been taking their drugs as prescribed. The diary is also a useful record for doctors who may see the patient at other centres. Physiotherapists work with the patients from the first posttransplant day and supervise their physical rehabilitation. Patients are encouraged to attend the gymnasium as soon as they are fit and have an appropriate exercise programme tailored for their needs. They are not discharged to intermediate care till the nurses, physiotherapists, and medical staff involved in their care are satisfied that they are emotionally and physically ready.

Monitoring for acute rejection

Acute rejection remains the most important problem in the first year after cardiac transplantation. The introduction of endomyocardial biopsies by Philip Caves led to early treatment of rejection; this revolutionised the management of cardiac transplant recipient in the 1970s.[2] The introduction of cyclosporin and the combination of this drug with azathioprine and steroids resulted in a marked improvement in one-year survival.[3] Rejection episodes in patients on cyclosporin therapy tend to be less severe than in those on azathioprine and steroids alone and deaths due to acute rejection have fortunately become rare. At Papworth all cardiac transplant recipients have "surveillance" biopsies performed weekly in the first month, fortnightly in the second month, monthly for about the next three months and approximately every 2–3 months till the end of the first year, by which time most patients are on stable doses of immunosuppression. The frequency of surveillance biopsies after the first three months is determined to a large extent by the number of rejection episodes the patient has suffered. Patients who have treatment for an episode of acute rejection are always rebiopsied in the next week or two to establish the efficacy of treatment.

When surveillance biopsies are done histological rejection is often seen in patients who are clinically well. It is vitally important, therefore, to have a threshold for augmenting immunosuppressive therapy. At Papworth we treat all patients whose biopsies are graded ISHLT 3 or 4 regardless of symptoms. Patients with a grade 2 biopsy are only treated if they have symptoms or signs of rejection.[4] With this policy we believe we avoid overtreating a large number of patients. Close links between the transplant physician and pathologist are vital to ensure optimal patient care and we have found it extremely useful, particularly when the biopsy appearances are atypical or when there is a possibility of sampling error.

Non-invasive monitoring

Although endomyocardial biopsy is safe in experienced hands, it is uncomfortable and complications are more frequent if the operator is less experienced. Various non-invasive methods of diagnosing rejection have been investigated over the last 10 years but none has gained widespread acceptability. Echocardiography concentrating on indices of diastolic function has been shown to be a sensitive indicator of rejection.[5] The technique is, however, operator dependent and requires a dedicated technician and machine to deal with the workload of a busy transplant unit. Echocardiography is particularly valuable in the paediatric population where invasive procedures often require general anaesthesia.

The earliest method of diagnosing rejection was based on the work of Lower and Shumway who found that the process was associated with a fall in the summated voltage of the R wave amplitude on a surface electrocardiogram.[6] With the introduction of cyclosporin into clinical practice, this method was found to be insensitive, probably because rejection in these patients is associated with less intercellular oedema. Monitoring evoked T-wave amplitude, late potentials, and evoked epimyocardial electrograms have all been investigated at different centres with some success.[7,8] Further study is, however, required before any of these techniques can be recommended for widespread use.

Monitoring immunosuppressive therapy

All patients have a blood count, renal and liver function, and trough cyclosporin level checked at each visit. A chest radiograph and electro-cardiogram are done at every visit and serum lipids checked periodically. The transplant physician must review the results of the blood tests and endomyocardial biopsy and make appropriate changes in immunosup-pressive therapy. Changes in therapy are documented on a treatment chart and the patient contacted by telephone by a nurse in the continuing care unit. Where appropriate, patients are also asked to have further blood tests done by the general practitioner and the results sent to Papworth for review by the transplant team.

Maintenance immunosuppression

Most centres worldwide have used so-called "triple therapy" as main-tenance immunosuppression. This consists of some combination of cyclosporin, azathioprine, and corticosteroids. Unlike many other centres, particularly in North America, the Papworth programme has always attempted to wean patients off steroids after the first three months. Patients who have episodes of rejection on ceasing steroids or who have impaired renal function necessitating low cyclosporin levels are maintained on prednisolone, the usual dose being 5 mg per day.[9]

At Papworth we aim for a trough cyclosporin level of 300–350 micrograms/l in the first month after transplantation, 250–300 micro-grams/l for the next three months, and 200–250 micrograms/l from then till the end of the first year. Patients with significant renal dysfunction may need to be maintained at lower trough levels. In some patients it may prove impossible to achieve adequate immunosuppression without significant nephrotoxicity.

Azathioprine is administered in a dose sufficient to maintain the total white cell count between 4 and 6×10^9/ml. The usual dose is 1–2 mg/kg per day. Prednisolone is commenced at the time of transplantation (at 1 mg/kg/day) and the dose rapidly tapered to the maintenance level of 0.2 mg/kg/day. Patients are continued on this dose for the first three months and if they have had no more than one episode of acute rejection, steroids are then tapered over the next months. The daily dose is decreased by 1 mg per week or fortnight and a cardiac biopsy performed after every 5 mg decrement in dose. Approximately 70% of our patients are weaned off steroids completely; of those who remain on steroids long term, the usual dose of prednisolone is 5 mg per day.[9]

Tacrolimus (FK 506) has been investigated extensively in liver and renal transplant patients,[10] most of the work in heart transplant recipients being at one centre where considerable success has been reported in treating refractory rejection and in reducing the need for steroids.[11] A randomised

135

multicentre study comparing cyclosporin with tacrolimus for maintenance immunosuppression found no difference between the two drugs in the number of episodes of rejection or in survival, though tacrolimus was associated with less hypertension and hyperlipidaemia.[12] Mycophenolate mofetil is another drug which has undergone extensive evaluation in liver and renal transplant recipients.[13] Trials in cardiac transplant patients are ongoing; in contrast to azathioprine, it has anti-B cell activity and it is hoped that it may delay the onset of "chronic rejection" which in the transplanted heart manifests as allograft coronary artery disease. Recent unpublished reports suggest a small but significant decrease in the number of rejection episodes compared to patients on azathioprine in a randomised controlled trial.

Treatment of acute rejection

Episodes of acute rejection are treated with intravenous methylprednisolone (10 mg/kg/day for three days) and oral prednisolone then augmented to 1 mg/kg/day tapering by 5 mg per day to the maintenance dose. Patients have an endomyocardial biopsy within the next week or two to check the efficacy of treatment. Patients who have an episode of rejection refractory to two courses of methylprednisolone or recurrent rejection (usually three or more episodes) are treated at our institution with rabbit antithymocyte globulin (RATG). Cyclophosphamide has anti-B cell activity, unlike azathioprine, and may be useful in treating patients with recurrent rejection. It is more toxic than azathioprine and therefore less suitable for long-term use. At Papworth we have usually been able to substitute azathioprine for cyclophosphamide after a rejection-free period.

Tacrolimus and mycophenolate may also be used to treat refractory rejection. Other drugs used in refractory rejection include methotrexate[14] and the anti-CD3 antibody OKT3.[15] Total lymphoid irradiation[16] and photopheresis[17] are other therapeutic modalities used in some centres to treat rejection when conventional therapy fails.

Prophylaxis against infection

Like most other programmes,[18] we use co-trimoxazole as prophylaxis against *Pneumocystis carinii* infection. The dose used varies between centres; at Papworth we use one tablet of single-strength co-trimoxazole a day and continue this for 6–12 months by which time the total amount of immunosuppression has been reduced significantly; patients are usually on 5 mg of prednisolone a day or less when co-trimoxazole is discontinued. If the dose of prednisolone is augmented for the treatment of acute rejection, co-trimoxazole is restarted. Patients who are allergic to co-trimoxazole are treated with inhaled pentamidine once a month.

Strategies for preventing cytomegalovirus infection (CMV) vary widely between centres. At Papworth we have not used any prophylaxis in heart transplant recipients (unlike lung transplants) until recently. A small study using intravenous ganciclovir for four weeks in mismatched patients (donor CMV positive, recipient CMV negative) showed no significant benefit, probably because the duration of therapy was not long enough. Evidence from trials in other groups of patients has suggested that more prolonged therapy may be effective[19] as clinical cytomegalovirus disease is usually seen after immunosuppression has been augmented to treat an episode of rejection. The availability of oral ganciclovir has made prolonged therapy practicable; further studies are required to estabish the place of this drug in prophylaxis. Other centres have used hyperimmune globulin with variable success.

Toxoplasmosis is another rare but important infection that may be transmitted along with the transplanted heart.[20] This has been abolished with the use of pyrimethamine (25 mg/day) along with folinic acid (15 mg/day) for the first six weeks after transplantation. More recently, there has been evidence that oral co-trimoxazole used in the prophylaxis of *Pneumocystis carinii* infection also protects against toxoplasma.[21]

Oral acyclovir is used to treat herpes simplex virus infection but we do not use it as routine prophylaxis in heart transplant patients. Patients with recurrent infection often benefit from maintenance low doses of acyclovir. Patients exposed to herpes zoster infection who have antibodies to the virus are treated with high-dose oral acyclovir and zoster immune globulin.

Patients are treated with amphotericin lozenges in the first few weeks after surgery as prophylaxis against candidal infection but we do not use long-term prophylaxis at our centre.

Hypertension

Hypertension is a frequent problem in transplant recipients (50–90%) and is mainly a result of cyclosporin therapy though steroid therapy is a contributory factor.[22] Hypertension is usually seen within the first six weeks after transplantation and most commonly persists thereafter. The mechanism is unclear but may include a decrease in the fractional excretion of sodium by the kidney, an increase in sympathetic tone and hence peripheral resistance and an imbalance between vasodilator and vasoconstrictor prostaglandins. Hypertension aggravates cyclosporin-induced nephrotoxicity. The most effective class of drugs in cyclosporin-induced hypertension is the dihydropirine calcium antagonists. The most common side effect of this class of drugs is peripheral oedema which can be marked in patients on cyclosporin. Alternative drugs include angiotensin-converting enzyme inhibitors, α-adrenoceptor antagonists and β-blockers. Renal function needs to be closely monitored when angiotensin converting enzyme (ACE) inhibitors are commenced, particularly in patients with preexisting renal impairment due to cyclosporin.

Gout

Cyclosporin causes hyperuricaemia and about a third of cardiac transplant recipients suffer from clinical gout. Long-term use of non-steroidal antiinflammatory drugs is contraindicated in patients with renal dysfunction but may need to be used for acute attacks. Allopurinol, a xanthine oxidase inhibitor, needs to be introduced under careful supervision because it inhibits the metabolism of azathioprine. We reduce the dose of azathioprine by 75% and monitor the patient's blood count fortnightly for at least six weeks. We have had patients present with severe pancytopenia when they have been started on high doses of allopurinol without a concomitant reduction in azathioprine dose.

Hyperlipidaemia

Many cardiac transplant recipients have preexisting hyperlipidaemia associated with coronary artery disease. Lipid levels are often normal at assessment for transplantation even in patients who are not on therapy because of severe heart failure. Steroid therapy following transplantation invariably leads to a rise in lipid levels while the effect of cyclosporin is variable. Programmes that discontinue steroids altogether usually find a significant decrease in lipid levels.[23] Although allograft coronary artery disease is believed to be immunologically mediated, conventional risk factors like hyperlipidaemia may contribute.[24] Our practice has been to treat patients who remain hyperlipidaemic after they are weaned off steroids. Most patients are treated with an HMG CoA reductase inhibitor (usually pravastatin which is not lipophilic); some patients with a low HDL level and high triglycerides are treated with fibrates.[25] Patients are asked to report new symptoms; very few patients have had to discontinue therapy because of side effects (usually myalgia occasionally associated with a rise in creatine phosphokinase). We have avoided bile acid-binding agents because of the risk of binding immunosuppressive drugs. A recent study has reported a lower incidence of rejection and coronary artery disease and increased survival in patients treated with high doses of pravastatin in the first year after cardiac transplantation.[26]

Renal dysfunction

Although cyclosporin has revolutionised organ transplantation, numerous adverse effects soon become apparent. Renal dysfunction is among the most prominent of these and affects all patients to some degree.[27] Patient in severe heart failure often have mild to moderate renal dysfunction and this is exacerbated by cardiopulmonary bypass and perioperative cyclosporin therapy. The immediate effects of cyclosporin on renal function are probably reversible if the drug is discontinued or the dose reduced.[28] However, even "therapeutic" doses of cyclosporin can lead to the insidious development of chronic renal dysfunction. With increasing survival among cardiac transplant recipients, this problem may be seen more frequently in the future. The mechanism of renal injury is probably arteriolar vasoconstriction and injury to proximal tubular cells.

Endstage renal disease requiring dialysis or renal transplantation has occurred in approximately 4% of our patients.[29] The level of preoperative renal dysfunction does not seem to correlate with the later onset of renal failure. Those patients undergoing renal transplantation have a reasonable outcome provided they are selected carefully. Patients with associated cardiac allograft vascular disease can occasionally be considered for combined heart and kidney transplantation. The median time to onset of renal failure in our patients is 67 months.

Patients on cyclosporin need regular follow-up with attention to changes in renal function. In stable patients after the first 6–12 months, a reduction in cyclosporin levels is usually safe. Patients who have few or no episodes of rejection can have their level reduced earlier. In patients with established renal dysfunction, our practice has been to aim for a trough cyclosporin level of about 100 micrograms/l and restart prednisolone at 5 mg per day as additional immunosuppressive therapy. With this regime, rejection has not been a problem we have encountered. Some centres have opted to discontinue cyclosporin and convert patients to an azathioprine and steroid regime. However, acute rejection and graft failure has been reported with this method; while this may be acceptable in renal transplant recipients, it is potentially fatal in cardiac transplant patients. We refer patients to a renal physician when the creatinine is persistently above 250–300 micromoles/l.

Malignancy

One of the inevitable consequences of long-term immunosuppression appears to be a higher risk of neoplasia.[30] This has proved to be the case in all organ transplant recipients irrespective of the immunosuppressive regime used. The risk in cardiac transplant recipients may be slightly higher than in renal transplant patients because of the higher doses of immunosuppressive drugs used. Evidence from large databases suggests that the incidence of cutaneous malignancy and lymphoma is increased significantly but that other common tumours are not more prevalent than in the general population.[31] Tumours may grow more rapidly in immunosuppressed patients and the prognosis is therefore worse. At Papworth malignancy has

139

affected approximately 10% of patients surviving more than three months from the transplant.[29]

Cutaneous malignancy was the most common tumour in patients treated with azathioprine and steroids (in the precyclosporin era) and remains an important problem in current practice. It has been suggested that a metabolite of azathioprine (nitromidazole) causes photosensitivity and cancer. Unlike the general population, most skin tumours in these patients are squamous cell carcinomas rather than basal cell carcinomas. Regular inspection of the skin and early reporting of new or growing skin lesions is important, as is avoidance of excessive exposure to the sun. Patients who have had significant skin damage from sun exposure in the past may be at higher risk. Suspicious lesions should be excised as soon as possible and material sent for histology to confirm the diagnosis. Multiple and recurrent tumours are not infrequent and can lead to unsightly scarring and the need for skin grafting. Metastatic disease is also believed to be more common than in non-immunosuppressed patients. In the Papworth programme cutaneous malignancy accounts for about a third of all tumours.

The tumour most commonly associated with cyclosporin-based therapy is lymphoma; this was relatively rare in patients treated with azathioprine and steroids. There appears to be a relation between the dose of immunosuppression and the risk of lymphoid neoplasia.[32] The use of multiple courses of lympholytic therapy (particularly OKT3) increases the risk of lymphoma significantly. It is thought that the Epstein–Barr virus (EBV) has an important role in the pathogenesis of this tumour but the exact relationship between infection with the virus and the development of lymphoma is unclear.[33] Primary EBV infection may be more likely to be associated with lymphoma but is uncommon in adult cardiac transplant recipients in the United Kingdom. Most of these tumours are histologically non-Hodgkin's lymphoma but we have recently seen two cases of typical Hodgkin's disease.

The presentation and clinical course of these tumours is variable. The term "lymphoproliferative disease" (LPD) is used to describe a form of the disease which typically presents early after transplantation, is polyclonal with regard to the immunoglobulin class expressed, and may be responsive to a significant decrease in the dose of immunosuppression without resorting to chemotherapy or radiotherapy. Acyclovir, which has activity against EBV, is believed to be an important adjunct in the treatment of this disease. Histology of the lesion does not differentiate between tumours that are likely to respond to a rejection in immunosuppression and those that require further therapy. Our approach has been to start oral acyclovir (800 mg five times a day), discontinue azathioprine, maintain prednisolone at 5 mg/day, and reduce the dose of cyclosporin to achieve a trough level of about a 100 micrograms/l. Tumours may regress partially or completely with this approach. In patients presenting with a large tumour mass (and usually with monoclonal proliferations) the above strategy alone does not usually suffice and systemic chemotherapy and/or radiotherapy is required as for lymphomas in the non-transplant population. The prognosis for the latter group is generally unfavourable. It is unclear whether the two groups of tumours are distinct clinical entities or whether they reflect different stages of the same lesion. Close liaison between haematologist (preferably one who has experience in dealing with neoplasia in organ transplant recipients) and transplant centre is vital. The only way of minimising the risk of development of lymphoma appears to be to use the lowest dose of immunosuppression consistent with maintenance of allograft function; in practice this is difficult because we do not have a marker of the efficacy of cyclosporin at the cellular level.

Osteoporosis

Over the last 15 years cardiac transplantation has been offered to older age groups and it is likely that osteoporosis will be a bigger problem in the future. While osteoporosis may be a particular problem in the post-menopausal female recipient, it is also seen in men because of the immobility associated with heart failure. The use of steroids after transplantation is the main reason for the development of clinical symptoms. In our experience it usually presents within the first 2–3 months after surgery and may be more common in patients receiving multiple courses of augmented steroid therapy for acute rejection. Osteoporosis can affect the quality of life significantly in transplant recipients and can interfere with rehabilitation after surgery. The use of hormone replacement therapy in postmenopausal females is probably the best form of prevention but may be difficult in the patient with heart failure who is often on warfarin to prevent thromboembolism. There appears to be no consensus on the best method of prevention in males or on the treatment in either sex. When possible, steroids must be discontinued or the dose reduced; unfortunately this is often not possible in the early months after tranplantation. We also use biphosphonates as therapy and most patients do notice a significant reduction in symptoms with time.

Contraception and pregnancy

Many male transplant recipients have fathered children with no apparent ill effects in the offspring. Patients must, however, be counselled if they have a genetic cause for their heart disease (i.e. hypertrophic cardiomyopathy) and must consider the consequences of their reduced life expectancy after cardiac transplantation (approximately 50% survival at 10 years). The situation is more complicated in the female patient, with a small risk to the child and a larger one to the mother.[34,35] The exposure to immunosuppressive drugs *in utero* seems to lead to an acceptably low incidence of foetal malformations; however, if the mother suffers a cardiac complication during pregnancy there may be a risk to the foetus. The increased blood volume of pregnancy and the inevitable changes in the immune system are more likely to pose a problem to the mother. Immunosuppressive drug levels may alter in an unpredictable manner, increasing the risk of acute rejection despite close monitoring. While female cardiac transplant recipients have certainly had successful pregnancies our policy is to advise patients to consider the consequences carefully.

Contraception is obviously important for the female recipient and our current policy is to recommend the use of the oral contraceptive pill. Pills containing progesterone alone may interfer with cyclosporin less but in practice, any preparation may be safely used provided cyclosporin levels are monitored when the pill is first commenced. The intrauterine contraceptive device may result in a higher incidence of infection and is best avoided.

Vaccination and travel

As for other immunosuppressed groups, it is recommended that these patients receive the influenza vaccine every year. Live virus vaccines are contraindicated; this includes yellow fever, oral polio, BCG, and measles/mumps/rubella. We do not discourage patients from international travel, except in the first year when episodes of rejection and infection are more common.

Unrelated illness and drug interactions

Most stable cardiac transplant patients tolerate non-cardiac surgery well. The transplant team must communicate with the other doctors involved in the patient's treatment so that immunosuppression is continued during such episodes. At Papworth we encourage patients to report intercurrent illnesses and to check with us before starting drugs prescribed elsewhere to avoid potentially dangerous drug interactions. The interaction of azathioprine and allopurinol has been described earlier; other important examples follow.

Antihypertensive drugs

Diltiazem, nicardipine, and verapamil increase cyclosporin levels significantly and appropriate dose reduction is required.

Antibiotics

Erythromycin increases cyclosporin levels, aminoglycosides potentiate nephrotoxicity, imidazole antifungal agents increase cyclosporin levels markedly. Rifampicin induces the hepatic enzymes that metabolise cyclosporin and can lead to dangerously low levels.

Anticonvulsants

Phenytoin is a hepatic enzyme inducer like rifampicin and has similar effects. Carbamazepine also reduces cyclosporin levels.

Non-steroidal antiinflammatory drugs

Potentiate the nephrotoxicity of cyclosporin.

Antiarrhythmic agents

Amiodarone increases cyclosporin levels by about 30%.

Conclusion

Despite the many problems that cardiac transplant recipients face, most enjoy an excellent quality of life for many years. The transformation in the lives of patients who undergo successful transplantation is remarkable. By tailoring immunosuppression to each patient's needs, the transplant physician can help to minimise the risk of some of the long-term complications. When complications do arise, early diagnosis and prompt treatment are vital. The major goal of the next decade must be to develop a strategy for delaying the onset of or preventing allograft coronary artery disease.

References

1 Hosenpud JD, Novick RJ, Breen TJ, Keck B, Daily P. The Registry of the International Society for Heart and Lung Transplantation: twelfth official report. *J Heart Lung Transplant* 1995;**14**:805–15.
2 Caves PK, Stinson EB, Billingham ME *et al*. Serial transvenous biopsy of the transplanted human heart. Improved management of acute rejection episodes. *Lancet* 1974;**1**:821–6.
3 Oyer PE, Stinson EB, Jamieson SW *et al*. Cyclosporin in cardiac transplantation: $2\frac{1}{2}$ year follow up. *Transplant Proc* 1983;**15**:2546–52.
4 Hutter J, Wallwork J, English TAH. The management of rejection in cardiac transplant recipients: does moderate grade rejection always require treatment? *J Heart Transplant* 1990;**9**:87–91.
5 Hsu DT, Spotnitz HM. Echocardiographic diagnosis of cardiac allograft rejection. *Prog Cardiovasc Dis* 1990;**33**:149–60.
6 Lower RR, Dong E Jr, Glazener FS *et al*. Electrocardiogram of dogs with heart homografts. *Circulation* 1966;**33**:455–60.
7 Grace AA, Newell SA, Cary NRB *et al*. Diagnosis of early cardiac transplant rejection by fall in evoked T wave amplitude measured using an externalized QT driven rate-responsive pacemaker. *PACE* 1991;**14**:1024–31.
8 Warnecke H, Schuler S, Goetze HJ *et al*. Noninvasive monitoring of cardiac allograft rejection by intramyocardial electrogram recordings. *Circulation* 1986;**76**:72–6.
9 Parameshwar J, Sharples L, Schofield P *et al*. Can steroids be successfully withdrawn in heart transplant recipients? *J Heart Lung Transplant* 1995;**14**(2);S85.

10 European FK506 Liver Study Group. Randomised trial comparing tacrolimus (FK506) and cyclosporin in prevention of liver allograft rejection. *Lancet* 1994;**344**:423–8.
11 Armitage JM, Fricker FJ, del Nido P *et al.* The clinical trial of FK506 as primary and rescue immunosuppression in adult cardiac tansplantation. *Transplant Proc* 1991;**23**:3054–7.
12 Taylor DO, Barr ML, Radovancevic B *et al.* A comparison of tacrolimus and cyclosporine based immunosuppression in cardiac transplantation. *J Heart Lung Transplant* 1997;**16**(1):72.
13 European Mycophenolate Mofetil Cooperative Study Group. Placebo-controlled study of mycophenolate mofetil combined with cyclosporin and corticosteroids for prevention of acute rejection. *Lancet* 1995;**345**:1321–5.
14 Olsen SL, O'Connell JB, Bristow BR *et al.* Methotrexate as an adjunct in the treatment of persistent mild cardiac rejection. *Transplantation* 1990;**50**:773–6.
15 Bristow MR, Gilbert EM, Renlund DG *et al.* Use of OKT3 monoclonal antibody in heart transplantation: review of the initial experience. *J Heart Transplant* 1988;**7**:1–11.
16 Kahn DR, Hong R, Greenberg AJ *et al.* Total lymphatic irradiation and bone marrow in human heart transplantation. *Ann Thorac Surg* 1984;**38**:169–71.
17 Constanzo-Nordin MR, Hubbell EA, Fisher SG *et al.* Short term analysis of heart transplant patients after a single treatment with photopheresis for moderate rejection. *J Heart Transplant* 1992;**11**(2):200.
18 Olsen SL, Renlund DG, O'Connell JB *et al.* Prevention of *Pneumocystis carinii* pneumonia in cardiac transplant recipients by trimethoprim sulfamethoxazole. *Transplantation* 1993;**56**:359–62.
19 Winston DJ, Wirin D, Shaked A *et al.* Randomised comparison of ganciclovir and high-dose acyclovir for long-term cytomegalovirus prophylaxis in liver transplant recipients. *Lancet* 1995;**346**:69–74.
20 Wreghitt TG, Hakim M, Cory-Pearce R *et al.* The impact of donor transmitted CMV and *Toxoplasma gondii* disease after cardiac transplantation. *Transplant Proc* 1986;**18**:1375–6.
21 Orr KE, Gould FK, Short G *et al.* Outcome of *Toxoplasma gondii* mismatches in heart transplant recipients over a period of 8 years. *J Infect* 1994;**29**:249–53.
22 Miller LW. Long-term complications of cardiac transplantation. *Prog Cardiovasc Dis* 1991;**33**:229–82.
23 Price GD, Olsen SL, Taylor DO *et al.* Corticosteroid-free maintenance immunosuppression after heart transplantation: feasibility and beneficial effects. *J Heart Lung Transplant* 1992;**11**(2):403–14.
24 Parameshwar J, Foote J, Sharples L *et al.* Lipids, lipoprotein(a) and coronary artery disease in patients following cardiac transplantation. *Transplant Int* 1996;**9**:481–5.
25 Parameshwar J, Roberts M, Wallwork J *et al.* Treatment of hyperlipidaemia after cardiac transplantation. *Br Heart J* 1994;**71**(S):95.
26 Kobashigawa JA, Katznelson S, Laks H *et al.* Effect of pravastatin on outcomes after cardiac transplantation. *N Engl J Med* 1995;**333**:621–7.
27 Myers BD, Ross J, Newton J *et al.* Cyclosporin-associated chronic nephropathy. *N Engl J Med* 1984;**311**:699–705.
28 Kahan BD. Cyclosporin nephrotoxicity: pathogenesis, prophylaxis, therapy and prognosis. *Am J Kidney Dis* 1986;**8**:323–31.
29 Parameshwar J, Schofield PM, Large SR. Long-term complications of cardiac transplantation. *Br Heart J* 1995;**74**:341–2.
30 Penn I. Cancer is a complication of severe immunosuppression. *Surg Gynecol Obstet* 1986;**162**:603–10.
31 Penn I. The changing pattern of post-transplant malignancies. *Transplant Proc* 1991;**23**:1101–3.
32 Hanto DW, Frizzera G, Gajl-Peczalska K *et al.* Epstein–Barr virus, immunodeficiency and B cell lymphoproliferation. *Transplantation* 1985;**39**:461–72.
33 Pagano S. Epstein–Barr virus: culprit or consort? *N Engl J Med* 1992;**327**:1750–1.
34 Muirhead N, Sabharwal AR, Rieder MJ *et al.* The outcome of pregnancy following renal transplantation–the experience of a single centre. *Transplantation* 1992;**54**:429–32.
35 Hunt SA. Pregnancy in heart transplant recipients: a good idea? *J Heart Lung Transplant* 1991;**10**:499–503.

9 Cardiac complications following cardiac transplantation

Janet M McComb

Introduction

Cardiac complications after cardiac transplantation may be considered as early or late: complications within the first few weeks are either due to arrhythmias, to a variety of surgical problems or to rejection, and late complications are most often the result of graft vasculopathy. Other complications of transplantation in general, e.g. hypertension, will have an impact on the heart and so are also relevant.

The transplanted heart is, of course, not normal, primarily because of denervation. These physiological abnormalities, e.g. sinus tachycardia, are expected after transplantation and are not pathological.

The ECG after cardiac transplantation

The heart rate is normally increased after transplantation,[1] presumably due to autonomic denervation, but tends to fall with time. It has been suggested that unusually high heart rates may be associated with an increased mortality.[1] The reasons for this apparent association are not clear. The increased heart rate may reflect impaired ventricular function and tachycardia-induced cardiomyopathy has been described in a cardiac transplant recipient.[2]

Recipient P waves, reflecting persistent electrical activity in the recipient atrial remnant, may be recorded on the surface ECG but are often inconspicuous during normal sinus rhythm. They are dissociated from the donor QRS complexes. They can cause diagnostic problems when there is donor bradycardia, with either AV block or sinus arrest.

Right bundle branch block is common, occurring in up to 70% of recipients.[3-7] It may be due to inadequate preservation of the right ventricle at the time of surgery and may reflect either raised right heart pressures[3] or right ventricular dysfunction.[4] although this is not an invariable association.[5] Right bundle branch block *per se* does not appear to have any long-term sequelae.[5]

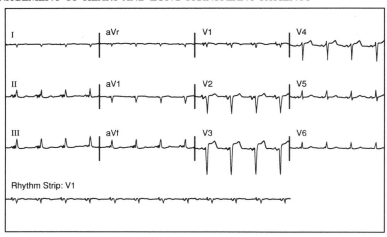

Fig 9.1   ECG from a transplant recipient.

Figure 9.1 shows a typical 12-lead ECG recorded from a transplant recipient.

Arrhythmias

Atrial arrhythmias

Atrial arrhythmias in the early posttransplantation period are common.[8-11] Atrial premature beats are frequent.[8,9,12] They are more frequent in patients with rejection[8] and decline with time in the first six months after transplantation.[8] Atrial tachycardia has been described in children in association with rejection.[13]

Atrial fibrillation may occur[8,11] and may be associated with subsequent mortality.[11] It can be treated with antiarrhythmic drugs such as propafenone or amiodarone or by cardioversion. Digoxin is thought not to be effective as its mode of action is thought to depend on its vagolytic function and in the early postoperative period the heart is denervated and so not susceptible to this mechanism of action. β-blockers should be avoided where possible, as the heart depends on circulating catecholamines to increase its cardiac output and β-blockers interfere with this.

Atrial flutter specifically has been described in association with cardiac rejection[8] and is probably an indication for biopsy. It can be treated by overdrive pacing or cardioversion.

Ventricular arrhythmias

Ventricular arrhythmias are also common, although less so than in normal hearts.[14] Ventricular premature beats are probably of no consequence,[8,14] although it has been suggested that they are related to subsequent mortality from transplant coronary disease.[12] They decline with time after transplantation.[8,9] Sustained ventricular arrhythmias, e.g. fibrillation or tachycardia, are rare, at least early after transplantation,[8,10] and in our experience have occurred mainly in association with the use of antiarrhythmic drugs for the treatment of atrial fibrillation. Late after transplantation, sudden cardiac death, presumably due to either ventricular fibrillation or asystole, is probably one of the more common modes of death and occurs in relation to graft coronary disease and acute coronary occlusion.

Other tachycardias

Rarely the transplanted heart may have an accessory pathway and be capable of sustaining a reentrant supraventricular tachycardia.[15] This is uncommon but if it occurs, it can be treated by radiofrequency ablation.[16] Other rare arrhythmias have also been described.[2,17]

Bradycardias

Sinus node dysfunction

Sinus bradycardia is common immediately after cardiac transplantation[10] and the heart rate may be supported either by isoprenaline or pacing, preferably atrial, or both. Bradycardia may persist for some time as sinus node dysfunction is quite common, occurring in up 64% early after transplantation[10] and in up to 29% of long-term survivors.[18] The prevalence of sinus node dysfunction varies from centre to centre, the reported requirement for permanent pacing varying from 4% to 29%.[10,19–22] The aetiology of sinus node dysfunction posttransplantation has not been clearly established but it has been suggested that it is due to abnormalities of the doctor sinus node[19] or to perioperative ischaemia.[21] One centre with a high pacemaker implantation rate for sinus node dysfunction[21] has shown a decline in pacemaker implantation with experience, suggesting a learning curve with improvements in surgical technique and a reduction in surgical trauma.[23]

Sinus node function improves with time after cardiac transplantation, even in those recipients with initially normal sinus node function.[24] This observation is supported by indirect evidence from those receiving pacemakers for sinus node dysfunction.[20,25,26] The requirement for pacing falls with time after transplantation, only 36% of those paced for sinus node dysfunction continuing to pace late after transplantation.[20,25]

Early after transplantation, when bradycardia is usual, theophylline can be used as a temporary positive chronotropic agent.[27,28] Intravenous aminophylline, however, improves markers of sinus node dysfunction but does not resolve the underlying abnormality.[29]

147

Permanent pacing is appropriate in transplant recipients with *symptomatic* sinus node dysfunction although, as discussed above, it may not be necessary in the long term.[20,25] The most appropriate mode of pacing for these patients has not been established. Although there is often chronotropic incompetence[30] there is little evidence that rate-responsive pacing improves exercise tolerance.[25] It seems reasonable to implant simpler rather than complex pacemakers, particularly as pacing may only be needed for a few months. Atrial pacing is probably more appropriate than ventricular pacing.

The need for permanent pacing in patients with *asymptomatic* sinus node dysfunction is less clear. These patients have often received pacemakers because of the risk of sudden death, despite the fact that these concerns are based on a single case.[31]

Permanent pacing does not seem to interfere with cardiac biopsy; although the permanent leads may be displaced by the bioptome, this actually rarely happens.[20]

Atrioventricular block

Although right bundle branch block is common, complete atrioventricular block is rare after transplantation. When it does occur, it usually requires long-term permanent pacing if it does not resolve within the first two weeks.[20,26,32] Dual-chamber pacing is probably the most appropriate mode, but any benefit of rate response has not been established.

Pseudoatrioventricular block is diagnosed when P waves on the surface ECG are dissociated from the QRS complexes, with the appearance of complete atrioventricular block, when the mechanism of bradycardia is in fact donor sinus arrest or bradycardia, the P waves being recorded from the recipient (Figure 9.2).[33]

Pericardial effusion

Pericardial effusion is quite common in the early posttransplantation period, occurring in up to 9% of patients.[34] It may be due to a size mismatch (recipient weight > donor weight),[34] the extra pericardial space allowing accumulation of fluid. While it may cause cardiac tamponade, it more commonly causes relatively minor haemodynamic embarrassment, with gradually deteriorating renal function. This may be sufficiently severe that pericardial aspiration is indicated. The effusion may be recurrent in up to one third and occasionally a pericardial window or pericardectomy may be required.[34] Rarely, the effusion may be infected, in which case surgical drainage with appropriate antibiotics is probably the best therapy.[35]

It is not surprising, therefore, that pericardial constriction may occasionally ensue, occurring in up to 1.5% of cardiac transplant recipients.[35]

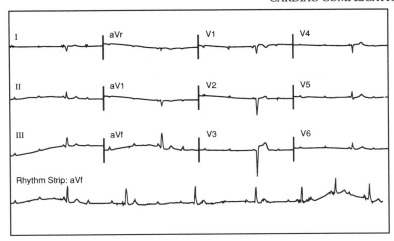

Fig 9.2   Pseudo AV block, showing P waves recorded from the recipient, and QRS complexes from the donor (note donor P wave just preceding second QRS complex on the rhythm strip, with different morphology from recipient P waves).

Figure 9.3 shows an echocardiogram demonstrating a pericardial effusion in a transplant recipient.

Heart failure

Heart failure after cardiac transplantation may be acute or chronic. The sudden onset of heart failure, either right or left, particularly early after transplantation, is usually due to cardiac rejection. It is therefore an indication for cardiac biopsy. It is treated in the usual way, with diuretics and inotropic agents. Right ventricular dysfunction is relatively common

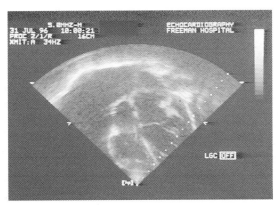

Fig 9.3   Echocardiogram showing a large pericardial effusion early after transplantation.

149

after transplantation and is due to one or more of the following: poor preservation, high pulmonary vascular resistance, size mismatch. A high filling pressure is required initially, to maintain cardiac output.

Chronic heart failure may either be the end result of cardiac rejection or due to recurrent myocardial infarction, following graft coronary disease. The patient, with perhaps silent ischaemia, may not notice infarctions and may present with either breathlessness or lethargy. It is treated in the usual way with diuretics, with or without ACE inhibitors. It may be an indication for reinvestigation and retransplantation.

The outcome of retransplantation is not as good as that of primary transplantation but nonetheless gives $55 \pm 8\%$ actuarial survival at one year and $33 \pm 8\%$ at five years (compared with $81 \pm 2\%$ and $62 \pm 2\%$ in those receiving primary transplants).[36]

Hypertension

Hypertension is common after cardiac transplantation, occurring in up to 75% of patients during long-term follow-up.[37,38] It is probably multifactorial and may be related to immunosuppressive therapy, i.e. cyclosporin and/or steroids. Overhydration and volume overload may be factors. It responds to dietary restriction of sodium.[39]

It is treated in the usual way, with ACE inhibitors (which may adversely affect renal function) and calcium antagonists (nifedipine causes gum hypertrophy and diltiazem spares cyclosporin). β-blockers should be avoided where possible. There was no difference in treatment with diltiazem or lisinopril,[40] both leading to improvement in up to two thirds of patients. As in non-transplant patients, left ventricular hypertrophy can regress with antihypertensive therapy.[41]

Myocardial infarction

Myocardial infarction may be quite common in long-term cardiac transplant recipients and occurs in relation to coronary disease. It may be silent, as the perception of anginal pain may be prevented by sympathetic afferent denervation. It presents, therefore, with heart failure or general malaise, weakness or arrhythmias. It is detected by the development of Q waves on the ECG and by the appearance of regional wall motion abnormalities, detected by echocardiography or radionuclide scanning. It is treated in the usual way, but patients will seldom present in time to benefit from thrombolysis and more often present late with heart failure. It may be detected on routine ECG and may have coincided with a two- or three-day period of lethargy. It may be an indication for coronary angiograpy, especially if retransplantation is being considered.

Graft coronary disease

Coronary artery disease is common after cardiac transplantation, being detected at routine coronary angiography in 44% at three years.[42] The angiographic appearance of the coronary lesions differs from that in ischaemic heart disease. There is diffuse concentric narrowing with distal vessel obliteration and poor development of collateral vessels.[43] Intimal thickness as detected by intravascular ultrasound increases progressively with time, up to 15 years after transplantation.[44] This accelerated coronary disease is the major cause of late morbidity and mortality after cardiac transplantation.[45] Myocardial infarction, congestive heart failure, and sudden death occur at a rate of 1.9% per year after the first year and account for a third of late deaths.[42] It is characterised by predominantly diffuse, concentric intimal proliferation in large and medium-sized epicardial arteries.[46] Angiographic findings include lesions identified in epicardial vessels or distal pruning.[43] These occur with a cumulative incidence of 10% per year. Pathologically it is a diffuse process, which can be detected by quantitative angiography or intravascular ultrasound.[47] After retransplantation, survival is lower,[48] with a repeat accelerated coronary disease recurring in up to 75%.[45]

Figure 9.4 shows two angiograms taken from the same patient demonstrating the angiographic appearances of graft coronary disease.

As the heart is denervated, angina is thought to be very uncommon (although it has been described in up to one third).[45]

It seems to predispose to thrombotic occlusion of coronary arteries, which may present as sudden death. It also causes acute myocardial infarction, which may be silent. Surveillance has traditionally been by routine coronary angiography, although whether this alters treatment in any way is doubtful. Non-invasive screening with exercise stress testing,

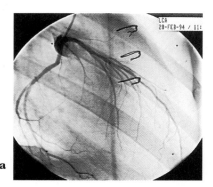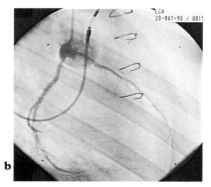

a   b

Fig 9.4a and b Left coronary angiography in the same recipient four years apart. Note irregularity, peripheral pruning, and paucity of vessels on the later film (figure b).

echocardiography, and perfusion scintigraphy has proved of limited value.[49,50]

The use of diltiazem may retard the development of coronary disease.[51] However, as the patients are asymptomatic, they do not routinely receive antianginal therapy (unless as antihypertensive agents). Discrete coronary stenoses detected at angiography may be treated with either angioplasty[52] or coronary artery bypass graft surgery.[53] Retransplantation is a rather unsatisfactory final choice of therapy.

Hyperlipidaemia

Hypercholesterolaemia is common after cardiac transplantation. Total serum cholesterol increases within six months of transplantation[54,55] and continues to do so progressively for at least two years.[54] Both statins and bezafibrate have been shown to reduce total and low-density cholesterol levels in transplant recipients,[56,57] although bezafibrate alone increased high-density lipoproteins[56] and simvastatin was shown to be better tolerated.[57] It has not yet been shown whether reduction in lipid levels has any effect on the development or progression of coronary artery disease in transplant recipients.

Biopsy-related complications
Coronary artery fistulae

These are a complication of repeated biopsy and as the septum is usually biopsied by choice, they most often affect the left anterior descending coronary artery.[58] They are detected at routine coronary angiography and

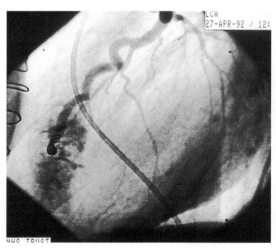

Fig 9.5 Angiogram showing a large coronary fistula persisting despite embolisation with coils.

are seldom large enough to cause haemodynamic consequences. Rarely, they can be sufficiently large to cause a shunt, leading to breathlessness. In such a case the fistula can be embolised with coils.

Figure 9.5 is a coronary angiogram of such a fistula.

Tricuspid regurgitation

Tricuspid regurgitation has been described and attributed to injuries induced at the time of endomyocardial biopsy and appears to be related to the number of biopsies.[59] It may be sufficiently severe to require valve surgery, either repair or replacement.[60]

References

1 Scott CD, McComb JM, Dark JH. Heart rate after cardiac transplantation. *Eur Heart J* 1993;**14**:530–3.
2 Ott P, Kelly PA, Mann DE *et al.* Tachycardia induced cardiomyopathy in a cardiac transplant recipient: treatment with radiofrequency catheter ablation. *J Cardiovasc Electrophysiol* 1995;**6**:391–5.
3 Gao SZ, Hunt SA, Wiederhold V, Schroeder JS. Characteristics of serial electrocardiograms after orthotopic heart transplantation. *Am Heart J* 1991;**122**:771–4.
4 Sandhu JS, Curtiss EI, Follansbee WP, Zerbe TR, Kormos RL. The scalar electrogram of the orthotopic heart transplant recipient. *Am Heart J* 1990;**119**:917–23.
5 Jessen ME, Olivari M-T, Wait MA *et al.* Frequency and significance of right bundle branch block after cardiac transplantation. *Am J Cardiol* 1994;**73**:1009–11.
6 Villa AE, de Marchena EJ, Myerburg RJ, Castellanos A. Comparisons of paired orthotopic cardiac transplant donor and recipient electrocardiograms. *Am Heart J* 1994;**127**:70–4.
7 Butman SM, Phibbs B, Wild J, Copeland JG. One heart, two bodies: insight from the transplanted heart and its new electrocardiogram. *Am J Cardiol* 1991;**68**:839–40.
8 Scott CD, Dark JH, McComb JM. Arrhythmias after cardiac transplantation. *Am J Cardiol* 1992;**70**:1061–3.
9 Little RE, Kay GN, Epstein AE *et al.* Arrhythmias after orthotopic cardiac transplantation. Prevalence and determinants during initial hospitalisation and late follow-up. *Circulation* 1989;**80**(suppl III):III-140–III-146.
10 Jacquet L, Ziady G, Stein K. *et al.* Cardiac rhythm disturbance early after orthotopic heart transplantation: prevalence and clinical importance of the observed abnormalities. *J Am Coll Cardiol* 1990;**16**:832–7.
11 Pavri BB, O'Nunain SS, Newell JB, Ruskin JN, Dec WG. Prevalence and prognostic significance of atrial arrhythmias after orthotopic cardiac transplantation. *J Am Coll Cardiol* 1995;**25**:1673–80.
12 Romhilt DW, Doyle M, Sagar KB *et al.* Prevalence and significance of arrhythmias in long-term survivors of cardiac transplantation. *Circulation* 1982;**66**(suppl 1):I-219–I-222.
13 Shreve MR, Crosson JE, Eusebio EJ, Braunlin EA. Electrocardiographic changes during long term follow-up of pediatric heart transplant recipients. *Am J Cardiol* 1993;**71**:1253–6.
14 Alexopoulos D, Yusuf S, Bostock J *et al.* Ventricular arrhythmias in long term survivors of orthotopic and heterotopic cardiac transplantation. *Br Heart J* 1988;**59**:648–52.
15 Goy J-J, Kappenberger L, Turina M. Wolff Parkinson White syndrome after transplantation of the heart. *Br Heart J* 1989;**61**:368–71.
16 Rothman SA, Hsia HH, Bove AA, Jeevanandam V, Miller JM. Radiofrequency ablation of Wolff Parkinson White syndrome in a donor heart after orthotopic heart transplantation. *J Heart Lung Transplant* 1994;**13**:905–9.
17 Rothman SA, Miller JM, Hsia HH, Buxton AE. Radiofrequency ablation of a supraventricular tachycardia due to interatrial conduction from the recipient to donor atria in an orthotopic heart transplant recipient. *J Cardiovasc Electrophysiol* 1995;**6**:544–50.

18 Bexton RS, Nathan AW, Hellestrand KJ et al. Sinoatrial function after cardiac transplantation. *J Am Coll Cardiol* 1984;**3**:712–23.

19 DiBiase A, Tse T-M, Schnittger I et al. Frequency and mechanism of bradycardia in cardiac transplant recipients and need for pacemakers. *Am J Cardiol* 1991;**67**:1385–9.

20 Scott CD, McComb JM, Dark JH, Bexton RS. Permanent pacing after cardiac transplantation. *Br Heart J* 1993;**69**:399–403.

21 Heinz G, Ohner T, Laufer G, Gasic S, Laczkovics A. Clinical and electrophysiological correlates of sinus node dysfunction after orthotopic heart transplantation. *Chest* 1990;**97**:890–5.

22 Miyamoto Y, Curtiss EI, Kormos RL et al. Bradyarrhythmias after heart transplantation. *Circulation* 1990;**82**(suppl IV):313–17.

23 Kratochill C, Schmid S, Koller-Strametz J et al. Decrease in pacemaker incidence after orthotopic heart transplantation. *Am J Cardiol* 1966;**77**:779–83.

24 Scott CD, Dark JH, McComb JM. Sinus node function after cardiac transplantation. *J Am Coll Cardiol* 1994;**24**:1334–41.

25 Scott CD, Omar I, McComb JM, Dark JH, Bexton RS. Long term pacing in heart transplantation is usually unnecessary. *Pace* 1991;**14**:1792–6.

26 Holt ND, Parry G, Scott CD et al. Permanent pacemaker use after cardiac transplantation: completing the audit cycle. *Heart* 1996;**74**:435–8.

27 Ellenbogen KA, Szentpetery S, Katz MR. Reversibility of prolonged chronotropic dysfunction with theophylline following orthotopic cardiac transplantation. *Am Heart J* 1988;**116**:202–6.

28 Redmond JM, Zehr KJ, Gillinov MA et al. Use of theophylline for treatment of prolonged sinus node dysfunction in human orthotopic heart transplantation. *J Heart Lung Transplant* 1993;**12**:133–9.

29 Rothman SA, Jeevanandam V, Seeber CP et al. Electrophysiologic effects of intravenous aminophylline in heart transplant recipients with sinus node dysfunction. *J Heart Lung Transplant* 1995;**14**:429–35.

30 Scott CD, Dark JH, McComb JM. Evolution of the chronotropic response to exercise following cardiac transplantation. *Am J Cardiol* 1995;**76**:1292–6.

31 Mackintosh AF, Carmichael DJ, Wren C, Cory-Pearce R, English TAH. Sinus node function in the first three weeks after cardiac transplantation. *Br Heart J* 1982;**48**:584–8.

32 Raghaven C, Maloney JD, Nitta J et al. Long term follow up of heart transplant recipients requiring permanent pacemakers. *J Heart Lung Transplant* 1995;**14**:1081–9.

33 Cataldo R, Olsen S, Freedman RA. Atrioventricular block occurring late after heart transplantation: presentation of three cases and literature review. *PACE* 1996;**19**:325–330.

34 Hauptman PJ, Couper GS, Aranki SF et al. Pericardial effusions after cardiac transplantation. *J Am Coll Cardiol* 1994;**23**:1625–9.

35 Carrier M, Hudon G, Paquet E et al. Mediastinal and pericardial complications after heart transplantation. Not-so-unusual postoperative problems? *Cardiovasc Surg* 1994;**2**:395–7.

36 Smith JA, Ribakove GH, Hunt SA et al. Heart retransplantation: the 25-year experience at a single institution. *J Heart Lung Transplant* 1995;**14**:832–9.

37 Ozdogan E, Banner N, Fitzgerald M, Musumeci F, Khaghani A, Yacoub M. Factors influencing the development of hypertension after heart transplantation. *J Heart Transplant* 1990;**9**:548–53.

38 Olivari MT, Kubo SH, Braunlin EA et al. Five year experience with triple drug immunosuppressive therapy in cardiac transplantation. *Circulation* 1990;**82**(suppl IV):276–80.

39 Singer DR, Markandu ND, Buckley MG et al. Blood pressure and endocrine responses to changes in dietary sodium intake in cardiac transplant recipients. Implications for the control of sodium balance. *Circulation* 1994;**89**:1153–59.

40 Brozena SC, Johnson MR, Ventura H et al. Effectiveness and safety of diltiazem or lisinopril in treatment of hypertension after heart transplantation: results of a prospective randomized multicenter trial. *J Am Coll Cardiol* 1996;**27**:1707–12.

41 Angermann CE, Spes CH, Willems S, Dominiak P, Kemkes BM, Theisen K. Regression of left ventricular hypertrophy in hypertensive heart transplant recipients treated with enalapril, furosemide and verapamil. *Circulation* 1991;**84**:583–93.

42 Uretsky BF, Kermos RL, Zerbe TR *et al*. Cardiac events after heart transplantation: incidence and predictive value of coronary arteriography. *J Heart Lung Transplant* 1992;**11**:s45–51.

43 Gao S-Z, Alderman EL, Schroeder JS, Silverman JF, Hunt SA. Accelerated coronary vascular disease in the heart transplant patient: coronary arteriographic findings. *J Am Coll Cardiol* 1988;**12**:334–40.

44 Rickenbacher PR, Pinto FJ, Chenzbraun A *et al*. Incidence and severity of transplant coronary artery disease early and up to 15 years after transplantation as detected by intravascular ultrasound. *J Am Coll Cardiol* 1995;**25**:171–7.

45 Keogh AM, Valantine HA, Hunt SA *et al*. Impact of proximal or midvessel discrete coronary artery stenoses on survival after heart transplantation. *J Heart Lung Transplant* 1992;**11**:892–901.

46 Johnston DE, Gao SZ, Schroeder JS, DeCampli WM, Billingham ME. The spectrum of coronary artery pathologic findings in cardiac allografts. *J Heart Transplant* 1989;**8**:349–59.

47 Pinto FJ, St Goar FG, Gao S-Z *et al*. Immediate and one year safety of intracoronary ultrasonic imaging. Evaluation with serial quantitative angiography. *Circulation* 1993;**88**(part 1):1709–14.

48 Karwande SV, Ensley RD, Renlund DG *et al*. Cardiac retransplantation: a viable option? Registry of the International Society for Heart and Lung Transplantation. *Ann Thorac Surg* 1992;**54**:840–44.

49 Smart FW, Ballantyne CM, Coconaugher B *et al*. Insensitivity of noninvasive tests to detect coronary artery vasculopathy after heart transplant. *Am J Cardiol* 1991;**67**:243–7.

50 Mairesse GH, Marwick TH, Melin JA *et al*. Use of exercise electrocardiography, technetium-99m-MIBI perfusion tomography, and two-dimensional echocardiography for coronary disease surveillance in a low-prevalence population of heart transplant recipients. *J Heart Lung Transplant* 1995;**14**:222–9.

51 Schroeder JJ, Gao SZ, Alderman EL *et al*. A preliminary study of diliazem in the prevention of coronary artery disease in heart transplant recipients. *N Engl J Med* 1993;**328**:164–170.

52 Halle AA, Wilson RF, Massin EK *et al*. Coronary angioplasty in cardiac transplant patients: results of a multicenter study. *Circulation* 1992;**86**:458–62.

53 Dunning JJ, Kendall SW, Mullins PA *et al*. Coronary artery bypass grafting none years after cardiac transplantation. *Ann Thorac Surg* 1992;**54**:571–2.

54 Stamler JSD, Vaughan DE, Rudd MA *et al*. Frequency of hypercholesterolemia after cardiac transplantation. *Am J Cardiol* 1988;**62**:1268–72.

55 Eich D, Thompson JA, Ko D *et al*. Hypercholesterolemia in long term survivors of heart transplantation: an early marker of accelerated coronary artery disease. *J Heart Lung Transplant* 1991;**10**:45–9.

56 Hidalgo L, Zambrana JL, Blanco-Molina A *et al*. Lovastatin versus bezafibrate for hyperlipidemia treatment after heart transplantation. *J Heart Lung Transplant* 1995;**14**:461–7.

57 Pflugfelder PW, Huff M, Oskalns R, Rudas L, Kostuk WJ. Cholesterol-lowering therapy after heart transplantation: a 12-month randomized trial. *J Heart Lung Transplant* 1995;**14**:613–22.

58 Locke TJ, Furniss SS, McGregor CGA. Coronary artery right ventricular fistula after endomyocardial biopsy. *Br Heart J* 1988;**60**:81–2.

59 Tucker PA, Jin BS, Gaos CM *et al*. Flail tricuspid leaflet after multiple biopsies following orthotopic heart transplantation: echocardiographic and hemodynamic correlation. *J Heart Lung Transplant* 1994;**13**:466–72.

60 Smith JA, Large SR. Tricuspid valve repair for tricuspid regurgitation after endomyocardial biopsy. *J Heart Lung Transplant* 1995;**14**:199.

10 General management of the lung recipient including aspects of postoperative shared care

Shinji Akamine and Tim Higenbottam

Introduction

heart-lung, single- and double-lung transplantations have been established as treatments for a wide range of endstage cardiopulmonary diseases such as primary pulmonary hypertension, cystic fibrosis, emphysema, idiopathic pulmonary fibrosis, and α1-antitrypsin deficiency.[1] The number of lung transplants, including heart-lung, single lung, and double lungs, has been at the rate of 1150 per year consistently in the last three years.[1] With enhanced organ preservation, operation techniques, immunosuppressive treatment, and diagnostic techniques for rejection and infection, the survival rate of lung transplantation has improved remarkably. However, approximately 30% of lung-transplanted recipients die in the early postoperative period. Risk factors for early death include infection and graft failure.[1,2] On the other hand, bronchiolitis obliterans (OB) is a common and often fatal complication of long-term survivors of lung transplantation.[3] The risk of OB is associated with a high frequency of acute rejection within the first three months after transplantation.[3] It is important for recipients of lung transplantation to be managed intensively during the early postoperative period. In this chapter, we review the general management of recipients of lung transplantation and discuss a developing treatment to improve survival.

History of lung transplantation

The first lung transplantation was carried out on a patient with chronic obstructive airways disease with a cancer. The patient died of renal failure 18 days after transplantation.[4] Combined heart-lung transplantation was first undertaken in a two-month-old infant with a complete atrioventricular canal defect. However, the patient died 14 h after transplantation as a result of respiratory failure.[5] Between 1963 and 1980, 38 patients received lung

156

transplantation but the median graft survival was only 8.5 days.[6] Only two recipients survived for six months and 10 months respectively after surgery. A third of patients had acute rejection contributing to graft failure and at least four had a problem with healing of the bronchial anastomosis.[6,7] At that stage, immunosuppressive treatment was based on azathioprine and prednisolone and was not sufficient to avoid rejection; moreover, steroids adversely affected the healing of the bronchial anastomosis. Other problems included perioperative care as well as surgical technique. Half of the patients died during surgery or within 10 days of surgery.

These problems were improved by the introduction of cyclosporin and better surgical procedures. Cyclosporin is an inhibitor of T cell-mediated immunoreaction,[8] which is remarkably effective in preventing the rejection of various organ allografts.[9] The efficacy of cyclosporin was proved for lung transplantation clinically as well as experimentally.[10] Cyclosporin not only has a superb immunosuppressive effect, but also reduces the dose of steroid and minimises the risk of insufficiency of bronchial wound healing.[11] In addition, the techniques of lung transplantation were improved by using an omental wrap around the bronchial anastomosis, which enabled protection and satisfactory revascularisation of the anastomosis,[12] and by transplanting heart and lung en bloc which provided better healing by converting collateral circulation from the coronary artery.[13]

In 1981, Stanford University initiated a clinical heart-lung transplant programme and performed the first successful heart-lung transplantation in a patient with primary pulmonary hypertension.[14] Following Stanford University, in March 1982 the University of Pittsburgh began a heart-lung transplant programme. In addition, in the UK, Harefield Hospital in 1983 and Papworth Hospital in 1984 started heart-lung transplantations. At present, 1954 heart-lung transplantations have been reported from 105 centres. However, the annual number of heart-lung transplantations has declined since 1989, in contrast to an increase in single and bilateral/double-lung transplantations.[1] In order to use the limited resource of donated organs fully, the indications for heart-lung transplantation have been changed.[15] For example, while initially primary pulmonary hypertension was indicated for heart-lung transplantation, recently it was reported that single lung transplantation for primary pulmonary hypertension is effective when there is no accompanying with heart dysfunction.[16]

Single-lung transplantation developed after heart-lung transplantation. The Toronto Transplant Group reported a successful single-lung transplantation performed in a patient with idiopathic pulmonary fibrosis in 1983, who survived more than five years.[17] This success was attributed to the immunosuppressive effect of cyclosporin and bronchial omentopexy. In 1986, a double-lung block was used to perform a double-lung transplantation in a patient with emphysema.[18] Early experience of *en bloc* double-lung

157

transplantation was associated with a higher frequency of airways complications compared with heart-lung transplantation. The delayed anastomotic healing was caused by poor blood supply, whilst the heart-lung block was compensated for by coronary bronchial bypass.[19] Therefore, the technique using two bronchial anastomoses was introduced to bilateral sequential-lung transplantations, which decreased the number of anastomotic complications.[20] In fact, the patients who underwent *en bloc* double-lung transplantation had a poorer survival than those with bilateral sequential-lung transplantation.[21] At the end of 1995, 3194 single-lung and 1845 bilateral/double-lung transplantations had been reported from a total of 124 lung transplant centres and the number is continuing to grow.[1]

Difficulties of lung transplantation

Lung allografts, compared with other solid organs, are the most difficult to control acute rejection. The reason is that the lungs contain a high dendritic cell population.[22] Therefore lung allografts are more vigorously rejected than hearts. In addition, acute lung rejection can occur in the absence of radiological abnormalities in the lungs[23] and moreover, the detection of acute rejection is difficult to distinguish from early post-operative infection in lung recipients because of the similar symptoms. Therefore, it is necessary to know not only the techniques of adequate immunosuppressive therapy and treatment of rejection but also the differential diagnosis of lung rejection and infection.

The lungs are the most easily infected of solid organs after transplantation because of many factors. The lungs are exposed to bacteria and viruses from the environment. In addition, immunosuppressive therapy with cyclosporin, azathioprine, and steroids creates conditions favourable for infection. Moreover, ineffective postoperative local mucociliary clearance[24] and breathing patterns may be related to denervation of the transplanted lungs and interrupted lymphatic and bronchial circulation. So, physiotherapy as well as prophylactic treatment for infection is required for postoperative management of recipients of lung transplantation.

One of the unique structures of the lung is the airway. In the early experience of lung transplantation, airway anastomotic complications were frequent and lethal.[6] Changing surgical techniques, such as telescoping anastomosis[25] and omental wrapping to cover the anastomosis (which is no longer practised[26]) and avoidance of excessive steroid,[27] decreased the number of the complications. In a recent review, the incidence of lethal airway complications was less than 3%[27] but the incidence of late complications of anastomotic stenosis which required stents[28,29] and laser[30] was approximately 10%.[27,31] The management of bronchial complications requires endoscopic skills including knowledge of endobronchial laser ablation and stent insertion techniques.

Pretransplantation

The pretransplantation management is an initial step to getting successful results. To begin with, recipients are those for whom transplantation is the only method of rescue. In addition, they should have a life expectancy of less than 18 months. Finally, the patient needs considerable enthusiasm and emotional resources and good family support.

Assessment for lung transplantation

Assessment for lung transplantation is important to ensure the maximum use of limited donor organs. In general, lung transplantation is indicated in patients with irreversible, progressive lung dysfunction, despite the use of medical treatments or surgical therapies. There are three procedures of lung transplantation – heart-lung, single lung and double/bilateral lung – and we have to ensure selection of the most beneficial procedure for the recipient.

Criteria for recipient selection (Box 10.1)

While this subject is dealt with in greater detail in Chap 2, it impacts on postoperative management. Patient selection should depend on predicted life expectancy. Because of the scarcity of the donor organs, many patients must wait for a long time and some of them die before transplantation. Therefore, a balance should be achieved in patient selection. The criteria for recipient selection may vary in each centre. The length of life expectancy will be indicated by the disability and progression of the original disease; generally, patients whose life expectancy is limited to less than 12–18 months should be enrolled on a waiting list. In Papworth Hospital, patients are assessed using the 12-min walk tolerance test.[32] A 12-min walking distance of less than 500 metres with a drop in arterial oxygen saturation below 80% indicates severe impairment of pulmonary function. Such individuals often require palliative or therapeutic oxygen. Arterial blood gas tension, particularly that of carbon dioxide ($PaCO_2$), is a good prognostic indicator of the severity of the pulmonary disease.

Primary pulmonary hypertension patients with a New York Heart Association functional class of III or IV, elevated mean right atrial pressure (> 20 mmHg), elevated mean pulmonary artery pressure (> 85 mmHg), decreased cardiac index (< 2 l/min/m^2),[33] and low pulmonary arterial oxygen saturation (SaO_2 $< 63\%$)[34] have a poor survival. In patients with chronic obstructive lung disease, the decline of lung function to below 30%, as shown by a predicted forced expiratory volume in 1 s (FEV_1), is suggestive of advanced lung disease.[35] In addition, the development of cor pulmonale and hypoxic hypercapnic respiratory failure are also indicators of poor prognosis.[36] Smoking after transplantation causes injury to allografted lungs so a potential candidate should stop smoking at least six months before referral.

Exclusive criteria have been changed considerably as experience of these procedures has improved. For example, initially patients with previous thoracic surgery such as sternotomy, pleurectomy or pleurodesis were excluded due to the high risk of postoperative bleeding.[37] However, such patients may be successfully transplanted with particular attention to haemostasis and use of aprotinin.[38] In another case, a patient with pulmonary hypertension with liver disease such as primary biliary cirrhosis may be considered for heart-lung/liver transplantation.[39] Systemic steroids can cause poor healing of the bronchial anastomosis[40] so the steroid dose was reduced preoperatively;[41] however, more recently, patients requiring steroids up to 0.3 mg/kg/day have been safely operated on.[42] Although some patients treated with conventional ventilation have had successful transplantation, the morbidity and mortality are still high in this group.[43]

Box 10.1 *Assessment of lung transplantation*

General
Life expectancy less than 18 months
Psychological and social stability
12-minute walk test <500 m with a drop in SaO_2 below 80%
No irreversible other systemic diseases
No contraindication to immunosuppression
No mechanical ventilation support
No active systemic infection such as aspergillus
No malignancy
No high-dose steroid therapy (<20 mg/day prednisolone)
Abstinence from tobacco >6 months
Required oxygen therapy

Age
<55 years (heart-lung, double/bilateral-lung transplantation)
<60 years (single-lung transplantation)

Parenchymal lung disease
FEV <30% of predicted value
DLCO <64% of predicted value
Evidence of cor pulmonale
Hypoxic hypercapnic respiratory failure

Pulmonary hypertension
Mixed venous oxygen saturation <63%
Cardiac index <1.5 1/min/m^2

Single or double/bilateral-lung transplantation
Not accompanied with bilateral septic lungs such as bronchiectasis and cystic fibrosis
Normal cardiac function
    Right ventricular ejection fraction >20%
    Left ventricular ejection fraction >40%

Therefore, because of the scarcity of donor organs and long waiting lists, such patients are not suitable for transplantation. As immunosuppressive therapy increases the risk of malignancy,[44] patients with a history of malignancy should be free from the disease for at least five years.[45] Insulin-dependent diabetes mellitus without complications is not a contraindication for lung transplantation. Patients with positive growth of *Aspergillus fumigatus* from sputum can be treated with aerosol natamycin and oral antifungal agents.[46] However, the presence of aspergilloma involving the pleura and/or chest wall remains an exclusion criterion, because intrathoracic infection cannot be cleared at the time of surgery. Moreover, potential aspergillus infection or colonisation should be avoided in single-lung transplantation, because single-lung recipients may develop more complicated infections than double-lung recipients after aspergillus infection.[47,48] Finally, patients for single or double/bilateral-lung transplantation should have normal cardiac functions, within general more than 20% of right ventricular ejection fraction[18] and more than 40% of left ventricular ejection fraction. Otherwise, patients with cardiac dysfunction can be selected for heart-lung transplantation.

Indications for heart-lung, single-lung, and double/bilateral-lung transplantation (Table 10.1)

The three primary indications for heart-lung transplantation are pulmonary hypertension, Eisenmenger's syndrome, and cystic fibrosis (Figure 10.1).[49] heart-lung transplantation requires one heart and both lungs from one donor. However, if the recipient is to be offered a single lung or bilateral lungs, the heart from the donor can be used in a cardiac transplantation. This is a more effective means of using limited donor organs. To this purpose, the "domino" procedure has been devised[50] in which the heart-lung recipient has a heart-lung transplant *en bloc* from a donor and then he or she donates his or her heart to another cardiac recipient.[51] This procedure not only makes best use of a limited source of donor organs, but has the added advantage that the donated heart does not suffer a neuroendocrine injury due to brain death. Moreover, the ischaemic time can be shortened.[52] Recently, the number of heart-lung transplants has declined. The reason may be that indications for heart-lung transplantation have been revised due to a shortage of donor organs. More than 50% of heart-lung transplant recipients have normal or near-normal hearts.[51] Therefore, the recipients who have a reversible cardiac dysfunction or repairable cardiac abnormality should keep their own heart.

The indications for single-lung transplantation are dominated principally by chronic obstructive lung disease,[49] such as emphysema, α1-antitrypsin deficiency, and idiopathic pulmonary fibrosis. Recently patients with primary pulmonary hypertension have been offered single or bilateral-lung transplantation.[53] Adequate right ventricular function can return rapidly and the grafted lung should restore the pulmonary vascular resistance. Grafted lungs with involved pulmonary oedema or pneumonia cause death.[16] No clear guidelines exist for selection for this form of surgery.[54] However, the patient with left ventricular failure and/or existing coronary arterial disease should be a candidate for heart-lung transplantation. Finally, candidates for single-lung transplantation should not have accompanying bilateral septic lungs such as bronchiectasis and cystic fibrosis.

The common indication for double/bilateral-lung transplantation is cystic fibrosis (Figure 10.1).[49] Pulmonary hypertension without cardiac failure may be an indication for double/bilateral-lung transplantation. Patients with emphysema and α-antitrypsin deficiency usually have a single-lung transplantation. Compared with fibrotic lung disease,[17] obstructive lung disease produced ventilation-perfusion imbalance after a single-lung transplantation[55] but this has not been confirmed by recent clinical studies.[56] Ventilation and perfusion scintigraphy showed the allograft had adequate ventilation-perfusion matching. However, the risk of over expansion of the remaining emphysematous lung led to compression of the transplanted lung and poor gas exchange.[57,58] In fact, single-lung recipients with emphysema required sequential-lung ventilation[57] or contralateral lobectomy[58] because of pulmonary dysfunction postoperatively.

Table 10.1   Indications for lung transplantation

Indication for transplantation	Type of procedure		
	HLT	BLT/DLT	SLT
Pulmonary vascular diseases			
Primary pulmonary hypertension (PPH)	+ +	+ *	+ *
Eisenmenger's syndrome	+ +	+ #	+ #
Chronic pulmonary thromboembolic disease	+ +	+ *	+ *
Pulmonary parenchymal diseases			
Idiopathic pulmonary fibrosis (IPF)	+ $	+	+ +
Cryptogenic fibrosing alveolitis	+ $	+	+ +
Sarcoidosis	+ $	+	+ +
Emphysema	+ $	+	+ +
α 1-antitrypsin deficiency (A1A)	+ $	+	+ +
Obliterative bronchiolitis	+ $	+	+ +
Pulmonary septic diseases			
Cystic fibrosis (CF)	+ + $	+	+ §
Bronchiectasis	+ $	+ +	+ §
Miscellaneous			
Lymphangioleiomyomatosis	+ $	+	+
Eosinophilic granuloma	+ $	+	+

HLT, heart-lung transplantation; DLT, double-lung transplantation; BLT, bilateral-lung transplantation; SLT, single-lung transplantation; + +, primary indication; +, alternative option; *, normal cardiac function; #, combined repaired cardiac abnormality; $, domino procedure; §, not accompanied by septic bilateral lungs

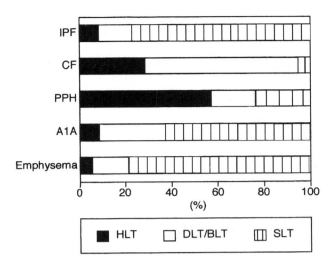

Fig 10.1   heart-lung (HLT), double/bilateral (DLT/BLT) and single-lung (SLT) transplantation indications by diseases (modified from the Registry of the International Society for Heart and Lung Transplantation in 1996[1]). For abbreviations, see Table 10.1.

Therefore, such patients may be considered for double/bilateral-lung transplantation.[59]

Management of recipients

Referrals for lung transplantation usually originate from pulmonary physicians. Adequate initial screening is essential to select appropriate recipients before an in-hospital evaluation. Screening should include diagnosis, age, medical treatments, cardiopulmonary functions, psychosocial status, and the presence of other systemic diseases and infections. The 3–5-day admission allows the patient to be extensively assessed.

Most centres have adopted a careful assessment procedure for prospective recipients of lung transplantation (Box 10.2). During admission, the patient also has an opportunity to meet other patients who have already received a transplant and to become familiar with all aspects of the transplant programme. The recipient and family are assessed by the transplant team (Box 10.3). At the end of the assessment, the team decides to accept the patient onto the transplant waiting list, to defer a final judgment and review after further information and settlement of unresolved issues, or to refuse the patient for transplantation. It is important to communicate with the refused patient and the referring physician about the results, so they understand the reasons.

163

When a candidate is accepted onto the waiting list, a transplant coordinator contacts the recipient. When a suitable donor is found the patient has a final general examination for surgery, including a chest X-ray, electrocardiogram, blood tests for haematology and biochemistry, and blood gas analysis, and then is given premedications for surgery.

Medical assessment and management

Most patients have been fully and appropriately investigated for their physical status by the referring physician. During admission, they are tested according to the assessment for transplantation (Box 10.2) which is conducted by the transplant staff. Routine examinations are performed for surgery. Tissue typing and virology are required. In particular, primary

---

Box 10.2 *Medical assessment for lung transplantation*

Routine examination
Haematology
Biochemistry, including renal and liver function
Coagulation screen
Antibody screening
Blood type
Tissue typing
Bacteriology
Virology
    Cytomegalovirus (CMV)
    Toxoplasma
    Epstein–Barr virus
    Herpes simplex virus
    Human immunodeficiency virus

Lung evaluation
Chest X-ray finding
Blood gases
Lung function test
Ventilation-perfusion scintigraphy
Pulmonary angiography
Right heart catheterisation

Heart evaluation
Electrocardiography
Echocardiography
Heart-catheterisation

Exercise test
12-minute walk test

Nutrition status

Psychopathology

Socioeconomics

Box 10.3 *Transplantation team*

Transplant surgeons
Chest physicians
Anaesthetists
Psychiatrists
Radiologists
Pathologists
Microbiologists
Transplant coordinators
Transplant nurses
   Intensive care unit
   Ward
Physiotherapists
Social workers
Occupational therapists
Pharmacists
Dieticians

CMV infection may be severe and usually fatal in CMV-negative recipients after lung transplantation.[60,61] In that case, prophylactic treatment is necessary to prevent CMV infection. In addition, if possible, mismatching of a CMV-positive donor and a CMV-negative recipient should be avoided to reduce the prevalence of CMV infection.

Medical management should be continued to maintain the condition of the recipient during the waiting period. When right heart catheterisation is performed, mainly in patients with primary pulmonary hypertension, we have seen the effects of prostacyclin infusion and inhaled nitric oxide administration. Long-term continuous prostacyclin infusion is effective not only in improving exercise tolerance, quality of life, and preventing dangerous syncope attacks, but also in enhancing life expectancy.[62] New treatments such as inhaled nitric oxide provide alternative therapies.[63] These treatments may be useful as a bridge to lung transplantation. In fact, long-term prostacyclin therapy prolongs the median time until death or heart-lung transplantation from eight to 17 months and doubles the chance of transplantation.[64] However, patients who do not respond to this treatment should continue to be considered for transplantation, because the improved survival with prostacyclin is not related to its immediate ability to cause pulmonary vasodilation. Therefore, such patients should also have the treatment while waiting for transplantation.[64] Inhaled nitric oxide may also be used as a therapeutic bridge to heart-lung transplantation for endstage primary pulmonary hypertension.[65] However, further studies are needed to clarify the duration and dose of inhaled nitric oxide therapy.

Patients with cystic fibrosis require the most specific management before and after transplantation. Cystic fibrosis is a multisystemic disease, which includes chronic bronchopulmonary infection, malabsorption, endo- and exocrine insufficiency such as diabetes mellitus, salt loss, meconium ileus equivalent, and liver disease. The secretions from the airways, including sinuses and nasopharynx, are a potential target for bacterial infection, mainly *Pseudomonas aeruginosa*, *Staphylococcus aureus*, and *Haemophilus influenzae*.[66] Therefore, patients with cystic fibrosis are treated with aggressive antibiotics against the bacteria during the waiting period.[67] Furthermore, diabetes mellitus must be controlled by insulin and mineral imbalance should be corrected. Because of malabsorption, patients with cystic fibrosis are malnourished and should be supervised by a dietician.

General care

During the waiting period, patients are helped towards a successful transplantation. They are engaged in a comprehensive programme that includes information and education about general aspects of transplantation. They can talk to the transplant staff and patients who have already received transplantation in the hospital, and can also be educated by the staff about preoperative rehabilitation, the need for donated organs, operative procedures, postoperative care, immunosuppression, rejection, and long-term outcome. Problems should be identified in exercise tolerance, medication, nutrition, social activity, and lifestyle.

Physiotherapy

In the UK, lung transplantation should be offered to patients who can achieve full rehabilitation to ensure maximum use of limited suitable donor organs. Under the direction of a physiotherapist, patients participate in a rehabilitation programme to achieve the best physical condition and functional level before and after transplantation. The programmes include treadmill walking and/or stationary bicycling. During exercise, patients are monitored for oxygen saturation, heart rate, and blood pressure. In addition, they learn an effective breathing pattern for thoracic surgery and pulmonary hygiene. Many patients have severe gas exchange abnormalities such as hypoxia, acidosis, and hypercapnia. However, once rehabilitation has started, the exercise capacity of the patient can be improved significantly.

Psychological support

Patients facing transplantation are nervous, with many concerns. Most of them fear for their lives when they realise that an organ is failing and they need organ transplantation. The problems they are concerned with include their own health, social status, perioperative care, rejection, long-term health, and financial stresses. For example, while the patients are on the waiting list, their own organ function is getting worse. It means they are going to die but in order to receive a donated organ, they are waiting for someone else's death. This is quite stressful. Psychiatrists should meet recipients and their families to help with their psychological problems. After transplantation, transplant recipients can start a new life but they will face complications such as graft rejection and the side effects of immunosuppressants. All transplant staff should be aware of the situation of the patient and explain the process of transplantation carefully when patients need more information about it.

In particular, the psychiatrist plays an important part in transplant programmes. The psychiatrist will meet with patients and their family to discuss any personal problems which they may have about the transplant process and help them to resolve these. When patients occasionally need medication, the psychiatrist will discuss this with the pharmacist, to avoid adverse interactions with other medications.

Transplant coordinator

The transplant coordinator plays a vital role in the general management of transplantation. While candidates are waiting, the coordinator keeps in touch with them and knows their condition and problems. When patients have any problems, the coordinator helps to solve them. When donor organs are available, the coordinator will contact a suitable recipient and then prepare for the transplantation.

Social worker, pharmacist, dietician

In the waiting period, the patients and their families have problems with activity, anxiety, and finance. A social worker advises them on these matters. The pharmacist enquires about the current medication of the patient and explains the necessity, dosage, and potential side effects of the drugs. The pharmacist can also educate patients about perioperative drugs, including immunosuppressive agents and antibiotics, and their monitoring after transplantation. Malnutrition can cause impaired wound healing and decrease resistance to infection due to depletion of serum protein and negative nitrogen balance. To avoid these problems, preoperative nutritional assessments are performed and nutritional status should be optimised before transplantation. In particular, patients with cystic fibrosis are in a malnourished condition. Therefore, candidates for transplantation should be advised by a dietician to achieve normal nutritional status and ideal body weight.

Posttransplantation (Box 10.4)

The principles of early postoperative management consist of early extubation within 18–24 h after surgery; maintenance of negative fluid balance; and early mobilisation. After surgery, the patient is nursed on the intensive care unit (ICU) and managed by transplant nurses. The care of the lung transplant recipient includes various aspects of critical management, including respiratory support, haemodynamic monitoring and

> **Box 10.4** *Principles of postoperative care*
>
> *Management*
> Early extubation within 18–24 h
> Maintenance of a negative fluid balance
> Early mobilisation
>
> *Monitoring*
> Graft function
> Extent of immunosuppression
> Presence of infection

maintenance, antibacterial and antiviral prophylactic agents, and immunosuppressive treatment. Reverse isolation is necessary to prevent infection. After 2–5 days stay in the ICU, the patient is usually returned to a surgery ward but kept in isolation from other patients for a further 4–7 days. During this period, patients are monitored for graft function, the extent of immunosuppression, and the presence or absence of infection. Simultaneously, they are encouraged to mobilise as soon as possible and individualised physiotherapy is started according to the patient's needs. Most patients without severe complications are then discharged from the transplant centre at about one month postoperation. Clinic visits are arranged initially once a week and then once a month. The physician should advise patients to report any new symptoms, such as fever, cough, dyspnoea, and a decrease of lung function in home spirometry.[68]

Intensive care (Box 10.5)

After stabilisation in the operating theatre, the patient is moved to the ICU. Reverse isolation is required and personnel entering the room should adhere to strict handwashing procedures and wear gown, gloves, and mask. The electrocardiogram (ECG) and haemodynamic pressures are monitored continuously. If needed, the patient is supported on a ventilator. Mediastinal and bilateral chest drainage tubes are attached to water-sealed low-pressure suction (<15 cmH$_2$0) and then the patient is covered with heating blankets. The patient is restrained to prevent dislocation of lines and tubes when he or she awakes from anaesthesia. After stabilisation in the ICU, portable chest X-ray, 12-lead ECG, and blood tests, including blood cell counts, coagulation test, electrolyte balance, and renal function, are performed. Frequent measurements such as vital signs (heart rate, respiratory rate, and body temperature), haemodynamic monitoring (arterial blood pressure, pulmonary blood pressure, central venous pressure, pulmonary wedge pressure, and cardiac output), and blood gas analysis are obtained. A 2:1 nurse:patient ratio is often necessary for the first day and then one-to-one nursing care is required.

Box 10.5 *Postoperative management*

Respiratory management
Tidal volume 10–12 ml/kg
Positive end-expiratory pressure (PEEP) 4–6 cmH$_2$O
Peak inspiratory airway pressure < 30 cmH$_2$O
Blood gas (FiO$_2$ < 0.6)
  PaO$_2$ > 80 mmHg
  PaCO$_2$ < 40 mmHg
Pulmonary toilet
  Soft suction tube two-hourly
  Fibreoptic bronchoscopic suction when atelectasis and/or infiltration shadow
Chest tube drainage
  < 15 cmH$_2$O suction on water sealed

Haemodynamic management
Central venous pressure < 10 cmH$_2$O
Mean arterial pressure > 80 mmHg
Mean pulmonary arterial pressure < 50 mmHg
Urine volume > 0.5 ml/kg/h
Haematocrit > 30%

Respiratory management

The management of the patient in the ICU is mainly performed by the transplant surgical team for some days, depending on the centre. However, the medical team, including transplant surgeons, anaesthetists, and chest physicians, meet once a day to review the patient's condition. The principles for ventilator setting are to maintain more than 80 mmHg of oxygenation at the lowest inspired oxygen (at least FiO$_2$ < 0.6), and at the lowest airway pressure (< 30 mmHg); 10–12 ml/kg of tidal volume is used. The positive end-expiratory pressure (PEEP) is set to about 4–8 cmH$_2$O. Sometimes a greater level of PEEP is required for maintaining oxygenation but it should be remembered that too high an airway pressure causes deterioration of bronchial anastomotic healing and barotrauma in the early postoperative period. Furthermore, in the single-lung transplant recipient with chronic obstructive lung disease, PEEP occasionally caused overinflation of the native lung and poor haemodynamic circulation due to mediastinal shift. Therefore, zero PEEP and lower volume ventilation are used. Alternatively, a double-lumen intratracheal tube is useful for sequential lung ventilation[57] when blood gases do not improve. Adequate pulmonary toilet is necessary to aspirate secretions from the lungs. A soft endotracheal suction tube is introduced into the trachea two-hourly. Aggressive insertion of the tube can cause injury of the anastomosis so when there is significant secretion from the lungs and/or consolidation, atelectasis, and infiltration shadow in the chest X-ray, a fibreoptic bronchoscope is necessary for suction of secretions or diagnosis of the shadow.

169

The standard weaning protocol can be used for lung transplantation. Usually, when a condition of less than 0.5 FiO_2, 80 mmHg of oxygenation is achieved in spontaneous breathing, the patient is subsequently extubated. It is important to perform fibreoptic bronchoscopy before extubation to evaluate bronchial anastomoses and the colour of the distal bronchus. After extubation,a close-fitting mask delivering 40% oxygen concentration is applied. Chest physiotherapists help the patient with breathing exercises, vibration, and percussion for removal of lung secretions. During the exercise, pulse oximetry for monitoring oxygenation and heart rate should be in place to detect any deterioration of the patient's condition.

Haemodynamic management

Continuous haemodynamic monitoring is applied by using an arterial line, central venous line, Swan–Ganz catheter, and urinary catheter. They are introduced in the operating theatre. The arterial pressures have to be kept to more than 80 mmHg to maintain bronchial arterial flow by using inotropic substances such as dopamine and/or dobutamine. Pulmonary arterial pressures vary according to the original disease. Prostacyclin can be effective for persistent pulmonary hypertension after transplantation for primary pulmonary hypertension. Recently, the efficacy of continuous inhalation of nitric oxide has been reported in patients with pulmonary hypertension and transient graft dysfunction after lung transplantation.[69] The volume of urine should be maintained at more than 0.5 ml/kg/h to prevent renal dysfunction due to cyclosporin. Transfusion of blood is necessary when the haematocrit is below 30%. The patient with no CMV antibody should be transfused with CMV-negative blood. It has to be remembered that fluid overload causes pulmonary oedema. In patients with heart-lung transplantation, nitroglycerin (generally 0.5 to 1.0 micrograms/kg/min) is used to prevent coronary vasospasm.

Management of early postoperative graft dysfunction (Box 10.6)

After lung transplantation, graft dysfunction may occur in about 20% of patients in the early postoperative period.[70] If oxygenation deteriorates, the cause should be detected by using chest X-ray, perfusion scintigraphy, echocardiography, and chest computed tomography. If the cause arises from pleural complications such as pneumothorax and pleural effusion and/or obstruction of bronchus by sputum or lung secretions, it can be improved by interventional treatments. Pulmonary venous stenosis caused by thrombosis should be treated immediately with an anticoagulant and/or thrombolytic treatment. If the treatments fail, reoperation should be carried out and the thrombus removed under cardiopulmonary bypass. However, prolonged graft dysfunction caused by pulmonary venous obstruction is rarely reversible. Occasionally, retransplantation may be required.[71] However, with the limitation of donor organ sharing, retransplantation should

---

Box 10.6 *Causes of early graft dysfunction and its management*

Pulmonary venous thrombosis and/or stenosis
Anticoagulant and/or thrombolytic treatment
Reoperation and pericardial patch reconstruction
Extracorporeal membrane oxygenation
Retransplantation

Pulmonary hypertension
Prostacyclin
Nitric oxide

Reimplantation response
Prostacyclin
Nitric oxide
Extracorporeal membrane oxygenation

Mediastinal shift in single-lung transplanted recipients with chronic obstructive lung diseases
Sequential-lung ventilation in single-lung transplantation
Extracorporeal membrane oxygenation
Lobectomy or pneumonectomy of contralateral lung

---

be the last choice for graft dysfunction. Reimplant response manifested by pulmonary hypertension, pulmonary oedema, and respiratory failure[72] may occur from reperfusion injury which causes pulmonary endothelial dysfunction.

Nitric oxide has recently been shown to be a vasodilator of the pulmonary artery. Nitric oxide can be useful for endothelial dysfunction after lung reperfusion and pulmonary dysfunction following lung transplantation.[73] Extracorporeal membrane oxygenation may be useful.[74,75] Overinflation of the native lung in single-lung transplantation in patients with chronic obstructive lung disease causes a mediastinal shift to the grafted lung and a deterioration of oxygenation. A double-lumen tracheal tube may be useful for sequential-lung ventilation.[57] Contralateral lobectomy or pneumonectomy after single-lung transplantation for emphysema could be alternative treatments for the overinflated native lung to release compression of a grafted lung.[58]

Management of pain

Another important aspect of management is pain control after surgery. Chest pain usually causes dyspnoea, sleep disturbance, and appetite loss. Use of morphine by epidural or intravenous administration is usually effective for pain associated with surgery during the early postoperative period. Pain related to thoracotomy continues for 1–2 months. In this period, physiotherapy and rehabilitation are important for recipients. During treatments, patients generally complain of chest pain. In addition, the chest pain is also accompanied by cough and expectoration of sputum. Therefore, use of oral analgesic agents is essential to perform the treatments.

Monitoring for infection and rejection

Chest X-ray

Chest X-ray is performed twice a day for the first week and then once a day during the second week and, thereafter, twice a week. Abnormalities in the chest X-ray on acute rejection consist of lung changes such as ill-defined perihilar and lower zone nodules and/or septal lines. Pleural effusion may also be seen, alone or with the lung changes. When infection or rejection is suspected, a chest X-ray must be performed immediately. However, the chest X-ray shows a normal appearance in 26% of cases of acute rejection during the first month after surgery and in more than 70% after the first month.[35] Therefore, suspicion of the diagnosis should be raised by the development of symptoms, abnormal physical signs, and reduction of lung function.

Lung function test

Daily pulmonary function tests are started within five days of surgery, using a handheld battery-operated spirometer.[76] The device can show the FEV_1 and the vital capacity (VC). At one week after operation, formal testing takes place in the laboratory, including VC, FEV_1, total lung capacity (TLC), and the single-breath carbon monoxide gas diffusion test (DLCO). It has to be remembered that, initially, FEV_1, VC, and TLC are reduced due to the results of transient changes after thoracic surgery, but increase progressively over the next 2–3 months. Therefore, continuing failure of FEV_1 and VC arising in the first few months after surgery may be a sign of rejection or infection.[77] By retrospective analysis of episodes of acute rejection or lung infection diagnosed by histological examination, we have been able to confirm that a 5% reduction in FEV_1 or VC is associated with these complications.[68] All patients are educated to measure and record lung function using home spirometry. A full lung function test is performed at discharge and then at three, six and 12 months or when respiratory symptoms or more than 5% reduction in FEV_1 occur.

Fibreoptic bronchoscopy (Box 10.7)

Fibreoptic bronchoscopy is a useful procedure for the management of patients after lung transplantation. Usually, chest physicians perform it but therapeutic bronchoscopy can also be carried out by surgeons, anaesthetists, and radiologists. It may be used for suction of sputum and inspection of anastomoses and when patients have suspected rejection or infection, bronchoscopy will provide histological, cytological, and biological materials from the transplanted lung by taking transbronchial lung

---

Box 10.7 *Utility of fibreoptic bronchoscope*

Investigation and therapeutic
 Suction of secretion
 Inspection of anastomosis
 Dilatation by balloon
 Laser ablation
 Insertion of silicon tube or self expanded metallic stent

Transbronchial lung biopsy
 Differential diagnosis between lung infection and rejection
  Histology
  Immunochemical histology

Bronchoalveolar lavage
 Cell counts (lymphocytes, macrophages, monocytes)
 Cytology (Immunocytochemistry)
 Culture (Microbiology)
 Supernatant

---

biopsies (TBLB) and bronchoalveolar lavage (BAL). The procedure can be performed easily and repeatedly with the patient receiving intravenous diazepam as sedation and local anaesthesia in the form of lidocaine.

TBLB are obtained from peripheral lung under fluoroscopic control by using the larger alligator forceps.[78] Currently, three biopsies are taken from each lobe of the lungs which show an abnormal shadow and should contain the three pulmonary anatomical elements including bronchial epithelium, alveolar, and blood vessel. Usually, five or six specimens are taken for diagnosis when an abnormal shadow is localised. Each biopsy specimen is fixed with 10% neutral formaldehyde and processed by use of a Shandon hypercutter. They can be processed within two hours in urgent cases. BAL is administered with two 50 ml aliquots of sterile normal saline at room temperature into infiltrated lobes as seen radiographically. In the case of a diffuse shadow, usually the saline is given to the left upper, lingula lobe or right middle lobe. Fluid is recovered by low suction into traps. The samples are separated into cellular components and supernatant and studied for cell counts, histology, cultured for microbiology, and immunocytochemistry.[79] In addition, when this procedure is performed urgently, it is important for quick diagnosis to contact pathologists, cytologists, and laboratory staff in advance. Finally, airway stenosis is one of the late complications of lung transplantation.[27] Interventional treatment for airway stenosis, such as dilation by balloon, laser ablation, and stent, can be performed under bronchoscopic inspection and fluoroscope.[30]

In our experience, complications were rare in 204 TBLBs and 30 studies of BAL in 52 heart-lung and lung transplant recipients.[80] Four patients developed minimal pneumothorax which was small enough not to require intercostal tube drainage and one suffered a severe haemoptysis requiring assisted ventilation for one hour. There was no other complication such as infection or excessive bleeding requiring a blood transfusion. However, it must be remembered that during the procedure, patients are monitored for heart rate and oxygenation by a pulse Doppler device to anticipate hypoxia or arrhythmia. A rapid decline of atrial oxygen saturation to below 80% is an indication to stop the procedure and withdraw the bronchoscope. If necessary, the patient should be sedated and intubated to enable assisted ventilation.

TBLB is routinely performed 10 days after transplantation, at the time of discharge from hospital, at three, six, and 12 months, and thereafter annually. TBLB is also carried out when a patient has suspected lung infection or lung rejection.[78] Currently, we are undertaking TBLB 2–3 weeks after treatment of acute rejection.

Immunosuppression (Box 10.8)

Immunosuppressive therapy is initiated when the recipient arrives at the hospital. The recipient is given 2 mg/kg azathioprine on arrival. Then, at induction of anaesthesia, 500 mg methylprednisolone is given by intravenous infusion and 50 mg rabbit antithymocyte globulin (RATG) is

---

Box 10.8 *Immunosuppressive regimens (in use at Papworth Hospital)*

Perioperative
  Azathioprine 2 mg/kg oral administration on arrival

Induction of anaesthesia
  Methylprednisolone 500 mg intravenous infusion
  Antithymocyte globulin (RATG) 50 mg/10 h drop infusion

Reperfusion
  Methylprednisolone 500 mg intravenous infusion

Postoperative
  Methylprednisolone 125 mg intravenous infusion at 1, 16, 24 h
  RATG 50 mg drop infusion day 1 and day 2
  Cyclosporin 4–6 mg/kg twice a day oral administration

Maintenance
  Azathioprine 2 mg/kg/day oral administration
  Cyclosporin 6–10 mg/kg/day oral administration
  Prednisolone 0.2 mg/kg/day oral administration

Acute rejection
  Methylprednisolone 1000 mg for 3 days intravenous infusion
  Prednisolone 1 mg/kg/day oral administration and tapered to 10 mg/day
  until improvement

---

administered by drop infusion over 10 h. At reperfusion, 500 mg methyl-prednisolone is administered intravenously followed by three doses of 125 mg methylprednisolone every eight hours. RATG is continued at a dosage of 50 mg/day on days 1–2 postoperatively. Cyclosporin 4–6 mg/kg twice a day is given orally as soon as the patient can take a diet. Oral maintenance immunosuppression consists of 6–10 mg/kg cyclosporin, ensuring a whole-blood trough level of about 400–600 ng/ml in the first five months after surgery, and then between 300 and 400 ng/ml with adjustment for renal function. Azathioprine is given at 2 mg/kg adjusted to keep the total white cell count at more than 4000 mm^3. More recently, a low dose of prednisolone has been introduced safely after surgery.[26] Antilymphocyte therapies are available commercially including ATG and OKT3 (a murine monoclonal antibody). During the anti-T cell therapy, the patient should continue to be "barrier nursed" under strict isolated conditions to avoid infection due to leucopenia. In addition, although OKT3 is a relatively safe therapy for acute rejection, antimicrobial prophylaxis must be considered when OKT3 is given.[81] However, RATG is no longer used perioperatively after cardiac transplantation in most centres and its role is under review after lung transplantation. Instead of RATG, IV cyclosporin 2–4 mg/h initially, adjusted to the high therapeutic level, is used as an alternative for the induction of immunosuppression.

During the first week after transplantation, blood levels of cyclosporin and white cell counts should be taken every day. In particular, patients with cystic fibrosis have malabsorption of cyclosporin so the dose may need to be high to maintain appropriate serum levels. An episode of acute rejection is treated with 500–1000 mg methylprednisolone intravenously for three days and an additional 1 mg/kg/day oral prednisolone followed by 10–15 mg/day tapering for two weeks. If the patient experiences two or more episodes of acute rejection, confirmed by lung biopsies, triple therapy is continued, consisting of cyclosporin, azathioprine, and low-dose (10–15 mg/day) prednisolone.

Infection

The lung is the most easily infected organ, not only after lung transplantation but also after other organ transplantation including bone marrow. There are several reasons for this situation after lung transplantation, including direct communication with the environment, denervated lung, anastomosis of the bronchus, impaired mucociliary function, immunosuppression, and bronchiolitis obliterans as a chronic rejection.[82] This is one of the problems and difficulties of lung transplantation.

Prophylaxis (Box 10.9)

Infections, including bacteria, fungus, virus, and protozoa, are common causes of morbidity and mortality after lung transplantation in the early

175

postoperative period.[2,83] Therefore, prevention of infection is important not only for the recipient but also for the donor lungs. The donor should be tested for cytomegaloviral antibody to avoid a mismatched transplantation. Even though there may be no evidence of pneumonia in the donor lungs, the lungs and airways are often injured by intubation or aspiration. Therefore, during the recipient procedure, trimmings from the resected bronchus or trachea are taken for microbiological tests and the bronchial tree is irrigated with normal saline. Preoperatively, prophylactic antibiotics, including an aminoglycoside and β-lactam agents such as an anti-pseudomonal penicillin or a third-generation cephalosporin, are commonly started and continued for at least 48 h. When the results of cultures from the donor trachea or bronchus are available, a more appropriate antibiotic regimen can be instituted. However, transmission of infection from the donor lungs was seen in only two cases from a total of 23 early infections.[84] Therefore, it is important to take frequent samples of sputum, urine, blood, and wound secretions for bacterial culture and to change to appropriate antibiotics.

CMV is the most common viral pathogen. A recipient negative for CMV antibody who receives an organ from an antibody-positive donor will have the most severe disease.[61] Therefore, prophylactic ganciclovir at a dose of

---

Box 10.9 *Prophylaxis for infection*

Bacteria
Aminoglycosides and the β-lactam agents
   Antipseudomonal penicillin
   Third-generation cephalosporin
   From induction of anaesthesia to 48 h postoperatively
Sensitive antibiotics against the cultured bacteria

Virus
Cytomegalovirus
   Donor positive/recipient negative
      Ganciclovir 5 mg/kg twice a day for 14 days
      Polyvalent immunoglobulin 50–100 mg/kg every week or every 2 weeks
      until seroconversion
   Recipient positive
      Ganciclovir 5 mg/kg twice a day for 14 days
Herpes simplex virus, donor or recipient positive
   Aciclovir 800 mg orally for 12 weeks

Protozoa
Pneumocystis carinii
   Trimethoprim 160 mg and 800 mg sulphamethoxazole twice a day, three
   times a week for ever
Toxoplasma
   Pyrimethamine 25 mg/day for 6 weeks

---

5 mg/kg twice a day is given for a period of at least 14 days to a CMV-negative recipient who receives CMV-positive organs. Moreover some institutes add polyvalent immune globulin for prophylaxis at a dose of 50–100 mg/kg every week or every two weeks. Prophylactic use of high-titre immunoglobulin may reduce the incidence of morbidity and mortality.[60] On the other hand, it has been reported that prophylactic ganciclovir failed to prevent CMV infection.[85] Further studies are necessary to prove the efficacy of ganciclovir. In such antibody-negative patients, serum specimens were tested to monitor of CMV-specific IgM by enzyme-linked immuno-sorbent assay (ELISA) to detect seroconversion.

Pneumocystis carinii pneumonia is one of the opportunistic infections which appears after transplantation due to immunosuppression. Without prophylaxis the incidence of the infection was reported in 88% of heart-lung transplantations.[86] Prophylactic treatment by trimethoprim 160 mg and 800 mg of sulphamethoxazole is applied to prevent infection from 2–3 weeks after transplantation for at least one year.[87] However, the therapy should be restarted if immunosuppression is augmented. An alternative treatment is aerosolized pentamidine.[88] For *Toxoplasma gondii*, pyrimetha-mine is reported to be efficacious in preventing the disease in antibody-negative transplant recipients receiving organs from antibody-positive donors.[89] Where this is not suitable due to side effects, 480 mg co-trimoxazole can be given orally.[90]

Fungal infections following lung transplantation are also major causes of morbidity and mortality.[48] Amphotericin B is still a first-line drug, but its potential nephrotoxicity makes its use problematic, especially with cyclosporin.[91] The prophylaxis of fungal infections in recipients of lung transplants has not yet been established. The introduction of fluconazole, itraconazole, and lipid-associated forms of amphotericin B offers promise for improving antifungal therapies.[92]

Management

There are four separate phases in infections after lung transplantation (Figure 10.2).[82,93] The immediate postoperative period is associated with bacterial and fungal infections, acquired during the operation or from donor organs. In the first three months, viruses such as CMV and herpes simplex virus transmitted from the donor organ and fungus acquired from the environment are associated with infections. After three months, viral and opportunistic infections such as *Pneumocystis carinii* appear. Finally, one of the major late complications is bronchiolitis obliterans, which is characterised as an obstruction of the small airways.[94] This provides favourable conditions for bacterial infection. Some patients with OB have died of accompanying lung infection.[83]

When recipients have symptoms such as fever, cough, increasing sputum, shortness of breath, and dyspnoea, infection should be suspected as well as rejection. Diagnosis is confirmed by transbronchial lung biopsies, bronchoalveolar lavage, and subsequent histology and microbiology and then the appropriate treatment should be performed according to the microbiologists's suggestions.

The treatment of bacterial infection should be based on the culture of samples and sensitivity testing. It is necessary to know the common pathogens of bacterial infections which include Gram-negative bacteria: *Pseudomonas aeruginosa, Serratia marcescens, Enterobacter* species, *Escherichia coli, Legionella* species, *Haemophilus* species, *Acinetobacter* species, *Klebsiella* species; and Gram-positive bacteria: *Staphylococcus* species, *Enterococcus,* and *Streptococcus pneumoniae.*[82] Sometimes antibiotics have to be given before the results of cultures are available. In such cases, initial treatment should comprise two agents at least, such as an aminoglycoside and β-lactam agents. The treatment should be continued until the patient has been afebrile for 72 h. If the patient still has a fever, an investigation of the origin of infection must be performed and appropriate antibiotics given. In addition, physiotherapy should be performed to prevent retention of bronchial secretions. Of course, if the fever continues for more than three days, a microbiologist must be consulted.

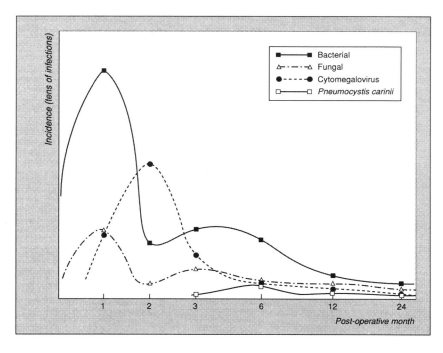

Fig 10.2 Timing of infections following lung transplantation (summarised from Kramer *et al.*[82] and Horvath *et al.*[93]).

Symptoms of CMV infection include general malaise, myalgia, abdominal discomfort, and fever, as well as leucopenia, thrombocytopenia, and atypical mononuclear cells in the blood. Definitive diagnosis is obtained by TBLB. In CMV infection, "owl's eye" inclusions are present in TBLB. CMV infection is treated intravenously with ganciclovir 5 mg/kg twice a day for 14–21 days[60] and in the case of severe pneumonia, CMV hyperimmune globulin can be added.[95]

Pneumocystis carinii pneumonia may be present with dyspnoea, fever, and cough but the pneumonia is not associated with production of sputum. Diffuse bilateral infiltrating shadow is seen on chest X-ray. TBLB and/or BAL is necessary to establish the diagnosis. In TBLB, foamy alveolar exudates are seen in which trophozoites can be demonstrated on silver stain. The drug therapy consists of a combination of sulphamethoxazole 100 mg/kg per day and trimethoprim 20 mg/kg per day. Usually, a clinical response is seen within four days.[96] Progressive deterioration after four days can be an indication for substituting pentamidine.

Fungal infections may arise from colonisation or latent infection in the airway of donor lungs or new opportunistic infection acquired following transplantation due to immunosuppression. Infection with aspergillus is not infrequent in lung transplantation.[48] Complicated aspergillus infections include aspergillus bronchitis, aspergilloma, pulmonary invasive aspergillosis, disseminated aspergillosis, empyema, and a retroperitoneal abscess. Transbronchial lung biopsy and/or bronchoalveolar lavage can be used to diagnose aspergillus infection. Amphotericin B is the only effective treatment for invasive aspergillus over 2–3 months but this is inevitably associated with irreversible renal dysfunction. A liposomal preparation of amphotericin B is available and can minimise renal toxicity.[92] Candida infection is not common, but *Candida albicans* often colonises mucous membranes, pharynx, and oesophagus. Under immunosuppressive conditions, candida may be pathogenic. Therefore, in the case of candida colonisation, prophylaxis by nystatin mouth wash and swallow may be given.

Rejection

Whilst the main cause of death in the early postoperative period is infection, rejection, especially chronic rejection which is manifested by pathological bronchiolitis obliterans (OB), is the major disability and cause of death among long-term survivors of lung transplantation. Acute rejection is usually reversible with treatment and rarely fatal. However, the frequency of acute rejection, particularly in the first three months after surgery, is the only predictor of bronchiolitis obliterans.[3] Therefore, control of acute rejection is fundamental to the management of recipients as well as control of lung infection and could enable reduction in the frequency of OB.

The first strategy is to diagnose rejection. It was initially thought that rejection of the heart and lungs would occur simultaneously. Therefore, endomyocardial biopsy (EMB) was substituted in the diagnosis of acute lung rejection. However, both experimental studies in baboons[97] and clinical heart-lung studies[98] suggested that lung rejection occurred without any evidence of cardiac rejection being detected by EMB. As the result, EMB has been abandoned[99] as a means of diagnosing lung rejection and TBLB was introduced to obtain lung tissue for histology.[78]

The second strategy is to decide when TBLB should be performed. It has already been made clear that both infection and rejection produce the same symptoms, physical signs, and laboratory data.[100] Moreover, rejection can occur in the absence of radiological abnormalities.[23] Therefore, we investigated a relationship between histological diagnosis and lung function during rejection and infection. We knew that lung function was changed by both events, notably FEV_1 and VC.[77] It is possible to use a small electronic turbine spirometer to record these measurements daily at home in order to detect early changes which can provide an indication for undertaking TBLB.[68] The use of this close monitoring has shown a reduction of lung function in the event of rejection.[101]

Finally, the last strategy is to differentiate rejection from infection. Acute rejection is characterised by perivascular infiltrates of lymphocytes, sometimes associated with similar infiltration of the small airway.[102] This is quite easily distinguished from the changes of infection.[78] The sensitivity of TBLB in diagnosing acute rejection or infection can be as high as 84%, with a specificity of 100%.[78]

Acute rejection

Acute rejection is observed as early as three days and as late as several years after transplantation. The average number of episodes is 3.5 times within one year. Acute rejection is associated with dry cough, dyspnoea, fever, breathlessness, and general malaise. These symptoms are also seen in infections. Physical examination often reveals a low-grade pyrexia, wheezes, and fine inspiratory crackles at the lung bases on auscultation. In addition, there may be an impairment of gas exchange manifested by a decrease in PaO_2 of more than 10 mmHg and a fall in FEV_1 and VC of more than 5%. Patients with acute rejection should have a chest X-ray and full respiratory function test at hospital. To confirm the diagnosis, TBLB and bronchoalveolar lavage should be performed. A standard classification and grading system has been formulated by the Lung Rejection Study Group.[103] After successful treatment, radiographic findings, lung function, and symptoms should improve. However, histological findings in TBLB 2–3 weeks after the treatment can occasionally be seen with persistent perivascular infiltration of lymphocytes.[104] In this case, we continue to treat with low-dose prednisolone.

Chronic rejection

Chronic rejection after lung transplantation is characterised by (OB), which is defined as an inflammatory disorder of the small airways, leading to severe airflow obstruction.[105] OB can occur as early as two months posttransplantation.[106] Most cases appear between 6–18 months after the transplant.[107] Various clinical series show that 43–62% of the long-term heart-lung transplant survivors and 25–31% of the single or double-lung transplant survivors have developed OB.[3,108,109] The causes of death are progressive respiratory failure and infection. The aetiology of OB has not yet been defined but potential risk factors, including HLA mismatching,[110] cytomegalovirus,[111] and frequent acute rejection,[3] have been proposed. We have found a strong correlation between the frequency and severity of acute attacks of rejection and the risk of developing OB.[101] Therefore we believe that control of acute rejection within three months may lead to the reduction of OB.

The diagnosis of OB is based on physiological and pathological aspects. A decline in FEV_1 of more than 5% at home spirometry can provide early detection of airway complications in the lungs. When OB is suspected, the pathological findings should be confirmed by TBLB. However, the sensitivity of TBLB for detecting OB is highly variable and, moreover, the specificity of the pathological diagnosis is low.[101,108,112] Therefore, when clinical symptoms and lung functions are compatible with OB and other causes are eliminated, OB should be the diagnosis. To this end, bronchiolitis obliterans syndrome (BOS) has been adopted to describe lung dysfunction after lung transplantation, recognising that there may or may not be pathologic evidence of OB present.[113] The BOS staging system is classified by the degree of impairment of lung function after lung transplantation (Box 10.10). BOS is also a major problem for medium to

---

Box 10.10 *Grading of bronchiolitis obliterans syndrome (BOS)*

0   No significant abnormality: $FEV_{1.0}$ 80% or more of baseline value

1   Mild BOS: $FEV_{1.0}$ 66% to 80% of baseline value

2   Moderate BOS: $FEV_{1.0}$ 51% to 65% of baseline value

3   Severe BOS: $FEV_{1.0}$ 50% or less of baseline value
    a. without pathologic evidence of bronchiolitis obliterans (OB)
    b. with pathologic evidence of OB

The baseline value is defined as the average of the two previous highest consecutive measurements, such measurements being obtained 3–6 weeks apart.

Excluding factors such as airway complications, infection, congestive heart failure, reversible airway reactivity, and systemic disease.

A significant decline in the $FEV_{1.0}$ will be determined by the average of two measurements made at least 1 month apart.

long-term survivors after lung transplantation and more than three episodes of acute rejection in the six months after transplantation is a sensitive prognostic indicator of subsequent functional decline.[114]

According to the results, the prevention of BOS is achieved by the control of acute rejection in the first six months. Triple regimens including cyclosporin, azathioprine, and prednisolone are given for maintenance of immunosuppression. Now, we need to revise this treatment for the maintenance of lung transplantation. Several new drugs such as cyclosporin G,[115] FK 506,[53] rapamycin,[116] 15-deoxyspergualin,[117] mycophenolate motefil,[118] leflunomide,[119] brequinar sodium,[120] and mizoribine[121] have been developed and used in clinical or experimental studies. FK 506 has been tried in patients with heart and lung transplants; the frequency of acute rejection is significantly lower than with cyclosporin.[122] It has been suggested that FK 506 may lessen the risk of BOS,[123] although this is not yet proved. FK 506 could be the first alternative agent to cyclosporin.

Chronic rejection has been treated by augmenting the immunosuppressive drugs with high-dose steroids,[124] azathioprine,[125] and antilymphocyte agents.[124] Beneficial results have been achieved with corticosteroids and the antilymphocyte preparations, but the relapse rate has been high after both therapies.[124] Some drugs (FK506,[123] mycophenolate mofetil,[126] rapamycin,[127] leflunomide[127]) may be used for treatment of OB. In particular, leflunomide has been developed not only as a novel immunosuppressive drug but also as an antiinflammatory.[128] Leflunomide used experimentally can inhibit chronic vascular rejection and BOS.[127]

Alternatively, a new approach to immunosuppressive therapy is required to prevent BOS. Simply increasing the dose of cyclosporin or oral steroids results in the major complications of opportunistic infection and renal failure. Therefore, targeted immunosuppressive treatment delivered to the transplanted organ may offer certain advantages; high topical dosage should be free of systemic complications. Inhaled nebulised steroid has been shown to be effective in preventing obliterative bronchiolitis in patients at risk after heart-lung transplantation.[129] In this study, patients at risk of OB with more than three rejection episodes in the first three months were randomised to nebulised budesonide 2 mg per day or to no treatment. This was given for one year along with conventional therapy. Follow-up was for three years. There was a slight difference in FEV_1 between the treated and untreated groups. Moreover, most of the patients in the group receiving budesonide were successfully weaned from oral steroids and they had fewer infections. Similarly, inhaled cyclosporin has also been reported to be more effective than oral administration with substantially lower blood levels.[130] In a non-randomised and uncontrolled trial, inhaled cyclosporin was added to conventional treatment in doses of 100–300 mg/kg and delivered by commercially available jet nebuliser.[130] Nine of 12 patients exhibited histologic resolution of five acute rejection and four chronic rejection episodes within three months of therapy.[131] New ways of targeting the immunosuppressive treatment could have specific advantages in the long-term therapy of lung and heart-lung transplant recipients.

We think that it is possible to identify different risk groups in patients developing BOS grade 1. We have studied the prognosis of 74 patients with BOS grade 1 retrospectively. The patients who had BOS grade 1 within two years, went on to suffer from BOS grade 2 or 3 later (87.8%) and died of OB. The five-year survival rate is significantly better in patients who fall to grade 2 after 60 days (64.3%) and patients who are still grade 1 or improving to grade 0 (83.1%) than in patients who fall to grade 2 within 60 days (26.4%). Patients who develop BOS grade 1 within two years and/or rapidly progress to grade 2 are at a high risk of early death of OB. This knowledge offers notions of new therapy to patients in high-risk groups.

Finally, if augmented immunosuppression fails and a continuous decline can be anticipated, retransplantation can be offered. However, in view of the lack of organ supply and the poor results of retransplantation,[132] it is now rarely performed as a treatment for OB.

Management of late complications

Airway complications

It is important to prevent airway complications. Unfortunately, when airway complications happen, management is very difficult. Bronchoscopic examination provides information on the state of the anastomosis. Major dehiscenses cause bronchopleural fistula and pyothorax which have a high mortality. Therefore, the only treatment for major dehiscenses is an operation for reanastomosis.[133,134] However, this is generally lethal as the patients develop sepsis and respiratory failure. Partial necrosis of the anastomosis is not usually fatal, but a stressful problem. In the early stages, partial necrosis causes mucosal ulceration which develops bacterial and fungal infections. Therefore, local treatments such as inhaled antibiotics are necessary to prevent an extensive pneumonia. The ulceration will be covered by epithelium, but the healing process causes stenosis. Narrowing of more than 50% requires treatment which consists of dilation by rigid bronchoscope or balloon, Nd:YAG laser ablation and stenting.[29,30] When persistent stenosis, malacia, and compression are observed, a silicon stent[135] or expandable metallic stent[136] may be required.

Lymphoproliferative disorders

Lymphoproliferative disorders are well known as Epstein–Barr (EB) virus-related cell tumours. The disorders occur in transplant patients who have a primary EB virus infection or a reactivated infection that results in uncontrolled proliferation of infected B lymphocytes in patients on cyclosporin treatment. In a healthy immunocompetent host, the EB virus infection follows a benign self-limiting course due to the generation of protective T-cytotoxic cells.[137] However, cyclosporin suppresses interleukin 2-mediated T cell proliferation, which impedes the defence mechanism. Withdrawal of immunosuppression, either alone or in conjunction with antiviral agents such as aciclovir or ganciclovir, produces prompt tumour regression, which is seen most often in patients who develop early lymphoproliferative disorders.[138] Alternative treatments include chemotherapy,[139] anti-B cell monoclonal antibodies[140] or immunoglobulin with or without interferon-$\propto$.[141,142] In the case of unresponsiveness and complications with compression and haemorrhage, surgical intervention may be required.

Physiotherapy and rehabilitation

Physiotherapy is begun within two hours after surgery to ensure early reexpansion of the lungs and to keep airways clear of secretions. In the intubated patient, airway suction is required every 3–4 h with postural drainage, tapping, and vibration to prevent atelectasis and pneumonia. Suction of airways must be careful to avoid any injury to the bronchial anastomosis. Moreover, hyperinflation of the lungs by using an Ambu-bag may lead to reduced bronchial flow and barotrauma. Therefore, airway pressure should be less than 30 cmH$_2$O. Oral or nebulised mucolytic agents can be useful to promote expectoration. After extubation, the physiotherapist may instruct the patient in the techniques of efficient breathing after thoracic surgery and the maintenance of aerobic capacity.

Exercise rehabilitation is started within 12–24 h after lung transplantation. During intubation, the patient requires passive muscular exercises, particularly to prevent deep vein thrombosis. Active exercises are introduced by sitting and standing, as soon as possible, usually within 48 h after surgery. In the next few days, the patient may walk accompanied by physiotherapists or nurses. During exercise, blood pressure, oxygenation by pulse Doppler, heart rate, and respiratory rate have to be monitored to maintain the oxygen saturation of the blood to a level greater than 90%. Usually, the patient can achieve the goal of his or her exercise capacity within one month. After discharge from hospital, the patient must continue the exercise programme.

Drug monitoring

After transplantation, pharmacists play an important role in managing not only immunosuppressive treatment but also antibiotic agents, vasoactive drugs, and respiratory medications. The dose of immunosuppression, such as cyclosporin, has to be decided by monitoring the blood level. A number of drugs affect the blood level of cyclosporin.[143] For example, diazepam, erythromycin, and ketoconazole increase its concentration and phenobarbitone, rifampicin, and intravenous sulphatrimethoprim decrease its concentration. In addition, cyclosporin can impair renal function and the effect is dose related.[91] Therefore, careful monitoring of blood urea, serum creatinine, urine electrolytes, and creatinine clearance is also essential. Some drugs, such as aminoglycosides, amphotericin B, sulphonamides, and trimethoprim, have a potential nephrotoxicity which can be increased with cyclosporin treatment. Renal dysfunction related to cyclosporin often recovers favourably by reducing the blood level of cyclosporin. Frusemide can be helpful. Azathioprine and steroids also have unfavourable side effects. High-dose azathioprine can cause myelotoxicity,[144] hepatotoxicity,[145] and carcinogenesis.[146] Corticosteroids may be associated with the development of a multitude of complications involving all organ systems.[147] It is very difficult to know all the interactions and side effects of these drugs so pharmacists should always be consulted by surgeons, physicians, anaesthetists, psychiatrists, and transplant nurses.

Finally, pharmacists may advise patients about all their medications including immunosuppressive agents, prophylactic antibiotics, antihypertensive drugs, and diuretics. Pharmacists should give information about the dose of each drug, methods of administration, potential side effects, and the reason for the prescription when patients are discharged from hospital.

General care (coordinator, psychiatrist, dietician, social worker, occupational therapist)

The coordinator will meet transplant recipients every day after transplantation and manage recipients' enquiries. If any problems occur, the coordinator will communicate with the person concerned.

After lung transplantation, the patient will face complications such as graft rejection and the side effects of immunosuppression. They can become anxious and depressed. The psychiatrist will meet the patient for discussion and will help them to resolve any problems. Occasionally, the patient will require medication and the psychiatrist will need to talk with the pharmacist to avoid adverse reactions with the immunosuppressants.

Usually after lung transplantation, oral intake is inadequate for only two or three days, if the patient does not have any complications. Therefore, special nutritional supports are not necessary for such uneventful patients. However, additional factors such as mechanical ventilation, infection, and fever may increase the patient's calorific requirements. Methods of nutritional supplement include the enteral or parenteral routes. Enteral nutrition is the more physiological route for nutrition. However, in such stressful conditions, paralytic ileus is frequently seen. In this condition, enteral nutrition causes abdominal fullness. Therefore, until enteral or oral nutrition is tolerable, parenteral nutrition may be given. During nutritional supplementation, total calorific intake needs to be measured daily and blood tests such as serum albumin, glucose, cholesterol, and triglyceride should be monitored to avoid metabolic complications including hyperglycaemia and hypoalbuminaemia. When complications occur, the dietician should be involved. Cholesterol and triglyceride must be monitored closely, because of the effect of cyclosporin.

Occupational therapists will help the patient with the practical aspects of his or her life at home. This will be done in cooperation with social workers. They will work with the patient and his or her family to coordinate the patient's posthospital care with regard to lifestyle, emotional support, physical practice, and rehabilitation for employment.

Education of patients (Box 10.11)

When the patient is discharged from hospital, he or she will need to be educated about lung transplantation in general, health care at home, and medical follow-up care. The patient should be aware of the symptoms and signs of rejection and infection and the side effects of prescribed drugs so that complications can be detected early. Furthermore, temperature, heart rate, lung function by home spirometry, new symptoms, and medications should be recorded daily and presented to the physicians. The patient should continue rehabilitation at home according to the pulmonary

---

Box 10.11 *Education for recipients of lung transplantation*

Basic knowledge
  Lung transplantation
  Immune system

Symptoms and signs
  Rejection and infection
    Acute, chronic, opportunistic infection
  Long-term complications
    Airway complication, lymphoproliferative disorders
  Side effects of medications
    Immunosuppressants, prophylaxis antibiotics

Medical follow-up care
  Rehabilitation
    Exercises and activity
  Nutrition
  Personal health surveillance
  Social activity

---

rehabilitation programme to promote mental and physical well-being and active life. The patient needs to be instructed in social and home activity. In the early postoperative period, it is recommended that the patient does not go to crowded places, use public transport, visit restaurants or meet anyone with respiratory infection. When the patient lives far from hospital, arrangements should be made with the local physician. Therefore, there should be frequent communication between the local physician and the transplant physician.

Conclusion

Human organ transplantation needs interdisciplinary medical team work. This includes surgeons, anaesthetists, physicians, microbiologists, psychiatrists, radiologists, pathologists, pharmacists, social workers, physiotherapists, occupational therapists, transplant nurses, and coordinators, as well as the technicians who manage cardiopulmonary bypass, immunological, and biochemical assays. Frequent team meetings are essential for good management of transplant recipients. Successful transplantation is a multidisciplinary achievement.

References

1 Hosenpud JD, Novick RJ, Bennett LE *et al.* The Registry of the International Society for Heart and Lung Transplantation: thirteen official report. *J Heart Lung Transplant* 1996;**15**:655–74.

2 Bando K, Paradis IL, Komatsu K *et al.* Analysis of time-dependent risks for infection, rejection, and death after pulmonary transplantation. *J Thorac Cardiovasc Surg* 1995;**109**:49–57.

3 Sharples L, Scott JP, Dennis CM *et al.* Risk factors for survival following combined heart-lung transplantation. *Transplantation* 1994;**57**:218–23.

4 Hardy JD, Webb WR, Dalton ML, Walker GR. Lung homotransplantation in man. *JAMA* 1963;**186**:1065–74.

5 Cooley DA, Bloodwell RD, Hallman GL *et al.* Organ transplantation for advanced cardiopulmonary disease. *Ann Thorac Surg* 1969;**8**:30–42.

6 Nelems JM, Rebuck AS, Cooper JD *et al.* Human lung transplantation. *Chest* 1980;**78**:569–73.

7 Veith FJ, Koerner SK. The present status of lung transplantation. *Arch Surg* 1974;**109**:734–40.

8 Borel JF, Feurer C, Gubler HU, Stahelin H. Biological effects of cyclosporin A: a new antilymphocytic agent. *Agents Actions* 1976;**6**:468–75.

9 Calne RY, White DJ. The use of cyclosporin A in clinical organ grafting. *Ann Surg* 1982;**196**:330–7.

10 Kamholz SL, Veith FJ, Mollenkopf FP *et al.* Single lung transplantation with cyclosporin immunosuppression. Evaluation of canine and human recipients. *J Thorac Cardiovasc Surg* 1983;**86**:537–42.

11 Saunders NR, Egan TM, Chamberlain D, Cooper JD. Cyclosporin and bronchial healing in canine lung transplantation. *J Thorac Cardiovasc Surg* 1984;**88**:993–9.

12 Lima O, Goldberg M, Peters WJ *et al.* Bronchial omentopexy in canine lung transplantation. *J Thorac Cardiovasc Surg* 1982;**83**:418–21.

13 Reitz BA, Burton NA, Jamieson SW et al. Heart and lung transplantation: auto-transplantation and allotransplantation in primates with extended survival. J Thorac Cardiovasc Surg 1980;80:360–72.

14 Reitz BA, Wallwork JL, Hunt SA et al. Heart-lung transplantation: successful therapy for patients with pulmonary vascular disease. N Engl J Med 1982;306:557–64.

15 Pasque MK, Trulock EP, Kaiser LD, Cooper JD. Single lung transplantation for pulmonary hypertension: three month hemodynamic follow-up. Circulation 1991;84:2275–9.

16 Bando K, Armitage JM, Paradis IL et al. Indications for and results of single, bilateral, and heart-lung transplantation for pulmonary hypertension. J Thorac Cardiovasc Surg 1994;108:1056–65.

17 The Toronto Lung Transplant Group. Unilateral lung transplantation for pulmonary fibrosis. N Engl J Med 1986;314:1140–5.

18 Patterson GA, Cooper JD, Dark JH, Jones MT. Experimental and clinical double lung transplantation. J Thorac Cardiovasc Surg 1988;95:70–4.

19 Lajos TZ. Noncoronary collateral blood flow. Ann Thorac Surg 1985;40:99.

20 Kaiser LR, Pasque MK, Trulock EP et al. Bilateral sequential lung transplantation: the procedure of choice for double-lung replacement. Ann Thorac Surg 1991;52:438–45.

21 Hosenpud JD, Novick RJ, Breen TJ, Daily OP. The Registry of the International Society for Heart and Lung Transplantation: eleventh official report. J Heart Lung Transplant 1994;13:561–70.

22 Prop J, Kuijpers K, Nieuwenhuis R, Wildevuur CRH. Why are lung allografts more vigorously rejected than hearts? J Heart Transplant 1985;4:433–6.

23 Millet B, Higenbottam TW, Flower CD, Stewart S, Wallwork J. The radiographic appearances of infection and acute rejection of the lung after heart-lung transplantation. Am Rev Respir Dis 1989;140:62–7.

24 Mancini MC, Griffith BP, Tauxe N. Assessment of mucociliary function in the tracheobronchial tree of the heart-lung transplant recipient. Surg Forum 1987;38:300–1.

25 Calhoon JH, Grover FL, Gibbons WJ et al. Single lung transplantation. Alternative indications and technique. J Thorac Cardiovasc Surg 1991;101:816–24.

26 Miller JD, de Hoyos A. An evaluation of the role of omentopexy and of early perioperative corticosteroid administration in clinical lung transplantation. The University of Toronto and Washington University Lung Transplant Programs. J Thorac Cardiovasc Surg 1993;105:247–52.

27 Shennib H, Massard G. Airway complications in lung transplantation. Ann Thorac Surg 1994;57:506–11.

28 Cooper JD, Pearson FG, Patterson GA et al. Use of silicone stents in the management of airway problems. Ann Thorac Surg 1989;47:371–8.

29 Higgins R, McNeil K, Dennis C et al. Airway stenoses after lung transplantation: management with expanding metal stents. J Heart Lung Transplant 1994;13:774–8.

30 Colt HG, Janssen JP, Dumon JF, Noirclerc MJ. Endoscopic management of bronchial stenosis after double lung transplantation. Chest 1992;102:10–16.

31 Date H, Trulock EP, Arcidi JM et al. Improved airway healing after lung transplantation. An analysis of 348 bronchial anastomoses. J Thorac Cardiovasc Surg 1995;110:1424–32.

32 McGavin CR, Artvinli M, Naoe H, McHardy GJ. Dyspnoea, disability and distance walked: comparison of estimates of exercise performance in respiratory disease. Br Med J 1978;2:241–3.

33 D'Alonzo GE, Barst RJ, Ayres SM et al. Survival in patients with primary pulmonary hypertension. Results from a national prospective registry. Ann Intern Med 1991;115:343–9.

34 Fuster V, Steele PM, Edwards WD et al. Primary pulmonary hypertension: natural history and the importance of thrombosis. Circulation 1984;70:580–7.

35 Bishop JM, Cross KW. Physiological variables and mortality in patients with various categories of chronic respiratory disease. Bull Eur Physiopathol Respir 1984;20:495–500.

36 Siassi B, Moss AJ, Dooley RR. Clinical recognition of cor pulmonale in cystic fibrosis. J Pediatr 1971;78:794–805.

37 Griffith BP, Hardesty RL, Trento A et al. Heart-lung transplantation: lessons learned and future hopes. Ann Thorac Surg 1987;43:6–16.

38 Kesten S, de Hoyos A, Chaparro C *et al.* Aprotinin reduces blood loss in lung transplant recipients. *Ann Thorac Surg* 1995;**59**:877–9.

39 Wallwork J, Williams R, Calne RY. Transplantation of liver, heart and lungs for primary biliary cirrhosis and primary pulmonary hypertension. *Lancet* 1986;**ii**:182–4.

40 Lima O, Cooper JD, Peters WJ *et al.* Effects of methylprednisolone and azathioprine on bronchial healing following lung autotransplantation. *J Thorac Cardiovasc Surg* 1981;**82**:211–15.

41 Patterson GA, Cooper JD. Status of lung transplantation. *Surg Clin North Am* 1988;**68**:545–58.

42 Schafers HJ, Wagner TO, Demertzis S *et al.* Preoperative corticosteroids. A contraindication to lung transplantation? *Chest* 1992;**102**:1522–5.

43 Massard G, Shennib H, Metras D *et al.* Double-lung transplantation in mechanically ventilated patients with cystic fibrosis. *Ann Thorac Surg* 1993;**55**:1087–91.

44 Rappaport DC, Weisbrod GL, Herman SJ. Cyclosporine-induced lymphoma following a unilateral lung transplant. The Toronto Lung Transplant Group. *Can Assoc Radiol J* 1989;**40**:110–11.

45 Grossman RF, Frost A, Zamel N *et al.* Results of single-lung transplantation for bilateral pulmonary fibrosis. The Toronto Lung Transplant Group. *N Engl J Med* 1990;**322**:727–33.

46 Heritier F, Madden B, Hodson ME, Yacoub M. Lung allograft transplantation: indications, preoperative assessment and postoperative management. *Eur Respir J* 1992;**5**:1262–78.

47 McDougall JC, Vigneswaran WT, Peters SG, Marshall WT, McGregor CG. Fungal infection of the contralateral native lung after single-lung transplantation. *Ann Thorac Surg* 1993;**56**:176–8.

48 Westney GE, Kesten S, de Hoyos A *et al.* Aspergillus infection in single and double lung transplant recipients. *Transplantation* 1996;**61**:915–19.

49 Goldberg M, Lima O, Morgan E *et al.* A comparison between cyclosporin A and methylprednisolone plus azathioprine on bronchial healing following canine lung autotransplantation. *J Thorac Cardiovasc Surg* 1983;**85**:821–6.

50 Sutor S, Wieczorek P, DeMaio K *et al.* Domino transplants. Sequential heart and heart-lung transplantation. *AORN J* 1988;**48**:876–89.

51 Smith JA, Cochrane AD, Esmore DS. Technique and results of cardiac transplantation using "domino-donor" hearts. *J Cardiac Surg* 1991;**6**:381–6.

52 Oaks TE, Aravot D, Dennis C *et al.* Domino heart transplantation: the Papworth experience. *J Heart Lung Transplant* 1994;**13**:433–7.

53 Starzl TE, Fung JJ, Venkataraman R *et al.* FK 506 for liver, kidney, and pancreas transplantation. *Lancet* 1989;**2**:1000–4.

54 Reitz BA. Adapted indications for lung transplantation: discussion report. *J Heart Lung Transplant* 1992;**11**:S286–S296.

55 Stevens PM, Johnson PC, Bell RL, Beall AC Jr, Jenkins DE. Regional ventilation and perfusion after lung transplantation in patients with emphysema. *N Engl J Med* 1970;**282**:245–9.

56 Trulock EP, Egan TM, Kouchoukos NT *et al.* Single lung transplantation for severe chronic obstructive pulmonary disease. Washington University Lung Transplant Group. *Chest* 1989;**96**:738–42.

57 Gavazzeni V, Iapichino G, Mascheroni D *et al.* Prolonged independent lung respiratory treatment after single lung transplantation in pulmonary emphysema. *Chest* 1993;**103**:96–100.

58 Le Pimpec Barthes F, Debrosse D, Cuenod CA, Gandjbakhch I, Riquet M. Late contralateral lobectomy after single-lung transplantation for emphysema. *Ann Thorac Surg* 1996;**61**:231–4.

59 Copper JD, Patterson GA, Grossman R, Maurer J. Double-lung transplant for advanced chronic obstructive lung disease. *Am Rev Respir Dis* 1989;**139**:303–7.

60 Gould FK, Freeman R, Taylor CE *et al.* Prophylaxis and management of cytomegalovirus pneumonitis after lung transplantation: a review of experience in one center. *J Heart Lung Transplant* 1993;**12**:695–9.

61 Wreghitt TG, Hakim M, Gray JJ *et al.* Cytomegalovirus infections in heart and heart and lung transplant recipients. *J Clin Pathol* 1988;**41**:660–7.

62 Dinh Xuan AT, Higenbottam TW, Scott JP, Wallwork J. Primary pulmonary hypertension: diagnosis, medical and surgical treatment. *Respir Med* 1990;**84**:189–97.

63 Pepke-Zaba J, Higenbottam TW, Dinh-Xuan AT, Stone D, Wallwork J. Inhaled nitric oxide as a cause of selective pulmonary vasodilation in pulmonary hypertension. *Lancet* 1991;**338**:1173–4.

64 Higenbottam TW, Spiegelhalter D, Scott JP *et al.* Prostacyclin (epoprostenol) and heartlung transplantation as treatments for severe pulmonary hypertension. *Br Heart J* 1993;**70**:366–70.

65 Snell GI, Salamonsen RF, Bergin P *et al.* Inhaled nitric oxide used as a bridge to heartlung transplantation in a patient with end-stage pulmonary hypertension. *Am J Respir Crit Care Med* 1995;**151**:1263–6.

66 Penketh ARL, Wise A, Mearns MB, Hodson ME, Batten JC. Cystic fibrosis in adolescents and adults. *Thorax* 1987;**42**:526–32.

67 Dinwiddie R. Management of the chest in cystic fibrosis. *J Roy Soc Med* 1986;**79**(suppl 12):6–9.

68 Otulana BA, Higenbottam T, Ferrari L *et al.* The use of home spirometry in detecting acute lung rejection and infection following heart-lung transplantation. *Chest* 1990;**97**:353–7.

69 Adatia I, Lillehei C, Arnold JH *et al.* Inhaled nitric oxide in the treatment of postoperative graft dysfunction after lung transplantation. *Ann Thorac Surg* 1994;**57**:1311–18.

70 Haydock DA, Trulock EP, Kaiser LR *et al.* Lung transplantation. Analysis of thirty-six consecutive procedures performed over a twelve-month period. The Washington University Lung Transplant Group. *J Thorac Cardiovasc Surg* 1992;**103**:329–40.

71 Dennis C, Caine N, Sharples L *et al.* Heart-lung transplantation for end-stage respiratory disease in patients with cystic fibrosis at Papworth Hospital. *J Heart Lung Transplant* 1993;**12**:893–902.

72 Sleiman C, Mal H, Fournier M *et al.* Pulmonary reimplantation response in single-lung transplantation. *Eur Respir J* 1995;**8**:5–9.

73 Date H, Triantafillou AN, Trulock EP *et al.* Inhaled nitric oxide reduces human lung allograft dysfunction. *J Thorac Cardiovasc Surg* 1996;**111**:913–19.

74 Aeba R, Griffith BP, Kormos RL *et al.* Effect of cardiopulmonary bypass on early graft dysfunction in clinical lung transplantation. *Ann Thorac Surg* 1994;**57**:715–22.

75 Glassman LR, Keenan RJ, Fabrizio MC *et al.* Extracorporeal membrane oxygenation as an adjunct treatment for primary graft failure in adult lung transplant recipients. *J Thorac Cardiovasc Surg* 1995;**110**:723–6.

76 Chowienczyk PJ, Lawson CP. Pocket-sized device for measuring forced expiratory volume in one second and forced vital capacity. *Br Med J Clin Res Ed* 1982;**285**:15–17.

77 Otulana BA, Higenbottam TW, Hutter J, Wallwork J. Close monitoring of lung function allows detection of pulmonary rejection and infection in heart-lung transplantation. *Am Rev Respir Dis* 1988;**137**:245A.

78 Higenbottam TW, Stewart S, Penketh A, Wallwork J. Transbronchial lung biopsy for the diagnosis of rejection in heart-lung transplant patients. *Transplantation* 1988;**46**:532–9.

79 Trulock EP, Ettinger NA, Brunt EM *et al.* The role of transbronchial lung biopsy in the treatment of lung transplant recipients. An analysis of 200 consecutive procedures. *Chest* 1992;**102**:1049–54.

80 Scott JP, Higenbottam TW, Clelland CA *et al.* A prospective study of 204 bronchoscopies in 52 heart-lung and lung transplant recipients using transbronchial biopsies. *Am Rev Respir Dis* 1990;**141**:A408.

81 Shennib H, Massard G, Reynaud M, Noirclerc M. Efficacy of OKT3 therapy for acute rejection in isolated lung transplantation. *J Heart Lung Transplant* 1994;**13**:514–19.

82 Kramer MR, Marshall SE, Starnes VA *et al.* Infectious complications in heart-lung transplantation. Analysis of 200 episodes. *Arch Intern Med* 1993;**153**:2010–16.

83 Chaparro C, Maurer JR, Chamberlain D *et al.* Causes of death in lung transplant recipients. *J Heart Lung Transplant* 1994;**13**:758–66.

84 Tamm M, Ciulli F, Dennis C *et al.* Early bacterial and fungal infections in lung transplantation. *Thorax* 1992;**47**:885–6.

85 Bailey TC, Trulock EP, Ettinger NA *et al*. Failure of prophylactic ganciclovir to prevent cytomegalovirus disease in lung transplant recipients. *J Infect Dis* 1992;**165**:548–52.

86 Gryzan S, Paradis IL, Zeevi A *et al*. Unexpectedly high incidence of *Pneumocystis carinii* infection after lung-heart transplantation. Implications for lung defense and allograft survival. *Am Rev Respir Dis* 1988;**137**:1268–74.

87 Kramer MR, Stoehr C, Lewiston NJ, Starnes VA, Theodore J. Trimethoprim-sulfamethoxazole prophylaxis for *Pneumocystis carinii* infections in heart-lung and lung transplantation – how effective and for how long? *Transplantation* 1992;**53**:586–9.

88 Nathan SD, Ross DJ, Zakowski P, Kass RM, Koerner SK. Utility of inhaled pentamidine prophylaxis in lung transplant recipients. *Chest* 1994;**105**:417–20.

89 Wreghitt TG, Gray JJ, Pavel P *et al*. Efficacy of pyrimethamine for the prevention of donor-acquired *Toxoplasma gondii* infection in heart and heart-lung transplant patients. *Transpl Int* 1992;**5**:197–200.

90 Wreghitt TG, McNeil K, Roth C *et al*. Antibiotic prophylaxis for the prevention of donor-acquired *Toxoplasma gondii* infection in transplant patients. *J Infect* 1995;**31**:253–4.

91 Myers BD, Ross J, Newton L, Luetscher J, Perlroth M. Cyclosporine-associated chronic nephropathy. *N Engl J Med* 1984;**311**:699–705.

92 Warnock DW. Fungal complications of transplantation: diagnosis, treatment and prevention. *J Antimicrob Chemother* 1995;**36**(suppl B):73–90.

93 Horvath J, Dummer S, Loyd J *et al*. Infection in the transplanted and native lung after single lung transplantation. *Chest* 1993;**104**:681–5.

94 Theodore J, Starnes VA, Lewiston NJ. Obliterative bronchiolitis. *Clin Chest Med* 1990;**11**:309–21.

95 Soghikian MV, Valentine VG, Berry GJ *et al*. Impact of ganciclovir prophylaxis on heart-lung and lung transplant recipients. *J Heart Lung Transplant* 1996;**15**:881–7.

96 Winston DJ, Lau WK, Gale RP, Young LS. Trimethoprim-sulphamethoxazole for the treatment of *Pneumocystis carinii* pneumonia. *Ann Intern Med* 1980;**92**:762–9.

97 Cooper DK, Novitzky D, Rose AG, Reichart BA. Acute pulmonary rejection precedes cardiac rejection following heart-lung transplantation in a primate model. *J Heart Transplant* 1986;**5**:29–32.

98 McGregor CG, Baldwin JC, Jamieson SW *et al*. Isolated pulmonary rejection after combined heart-lung transplantation. *J Thorac Cardiovasc Surg* 1985;**90**:623–6.

99 Higenbottam TW, Hutter JA, Stewart S, Wallwork J. Transbronchial biopsy has eliminated the need for endomyocardial biopsy in heart-lung recipients. *J Heart Transplant* 1988;**7**:435–9.

100 Penketh AR, Higenbottam TW, Hutter *et al*. Clinical experience in the management of pulmonary opportunist infection and rejection in recipients of heart-lung transplants. *Thorax* 1988;**43**:762–9.

101 Scott JP, Higenbottam TW, Clelland CA *et al*. Natural history of chronic rejection in heart-lung transplant recipients. *J Heart Transplant* 1990;**9**:510–15.

102 Hutter JA, Stewart S, Higenbottam TW, Scott JP, Wallwork J. Histologic changes in heart-lung transplant recipients during rejection episodes and at routine biopsy. *J Heart Transplant* 1988;**7**:440–4.

103 Yousem SA, Berry GJ, Cagle PT *et al*. Revision of the 1990 working formulation for the classification of pulmonary allograft rejection: Lung Rejection Study Group. *J Heart Lung Transplant* 1996;**15**:1–15.

104 Clelland CA, Higenbottam, TW, Stewart S, Scott JP, Wallwork J. The histological changes in transbronchial biopsy after treatment of acute rejection in heart-lung transplant recipients. *J Pathol* 1990;**161**:105–12.

105 Burke CM, Theodore J, Baldwin J *et al*. Twenty-eight cases of human heart-lung transplantation. *Lancet* 1986;**1**:517–19.

106 Burke CM, Theodore J, Dawkins KD *et al*. Post transplant obliterative bronchiolitis and other late lung sequelae in human heart-lung transplantation. *Chest* 1984;**86**:824–9.

107 Kramer MR. Bronchiolitis obliterans following heart-lung and lung transplantation. *Respir Med* 1994;**88**:9–15.

108 Kramer MR, Stoehr C, Whang JL *et al*. The diagnosis of obliterative bronchiolitis after heart-lung and lung transplantation: low yield of transbronchial lung biopsy. *J Heart Lung Transplant* 1993;**12**:675–81.

109 Chamberlain D, Maurer J, Chaparro C, Idolor L. Evaluation of transbronchial lung biopsy specimens in the diagnosis of bronchiolitis obliterans after lung transplantation. *J Heart Lung Transplant* 1994;13:963–71.

110 Harjula A, Baldwin J, Glanville A *et al.* Human leucocyte antigen compatibility in heart-lung transplantation. *J Heart Transplant* 1987;6:162–6.

111 Keenan RJ, Lega M, Dummer SJ *et al.* Cytomegalovirus serologic status and postoperative infection correlated with risk of developing chronic rejection after pulmonary transplantation. *Transplantation* 1991;51:433–8.

112 Yousem SA, Paradis IL, Dauber JH, Griffith BP. Efficacy of transbronchial lung biopsy in the diagnosis of bronchiolitis obliterans in heart-lung transplant recipients. *Transplantation* 1989;47:893–5.

113 Cooper JD, Billingham M, Egan T *et al.* A working formulation for the standardization of nomenclature and for clinical staging of chronic dysfunction in lung allografts. *J Heart Lung Transplant* 1993;12:713–16.

114 Sharples LD, Tamm M, McNeil K *et al.* Development of bronchiolitis obliterans syndrome in recipients of heart-lung transplantation – early risk factors. *Transplantation* 1996;61:560–6.

115 Copeland KR, Yatscoff RW. The isolation, structural characterization, and immunosuppressive activity of cyclosporin G (NVa2-cyclosporine) metabolites. *Ther Drug Monitor* 1991;13:281–8.

116 Kahan BD, Chang JY, Sehgal SN. Preclinical evaluation of a new potent immunosuppressive agent, rapamycin. *Transplantation* 1991;52:185–91.

117 Amemiya H, Suzuki S, Ota K *et al.* A novel rescue drug, 15-deoxyspergualin. First clinical trials for recurrent graft rejection in renal recipients. *Transplantation* 1990;49:337–43.

118 Taylor DO, Ensley RD, Olsen SL, Dunn D, Renlund DG. Mycophenolate mofetil (RS-61443): preclinical, clinical, and three-year experience in heart transplantation. *J Heart Lung Transplant* 1994;13:571–82.

119 Williams JW, Xiao F, Foster P *et al.* Leflunomide in experimental transplantation. Control of rejection and alloantibody production, reversal of acute rejection, and interaction with cyclosporine. *Transplantation* 1994;57:1223–31.

120 Cramer DV, Chapman FA, Makowka L. The use of brequinar sodium for transplantation. *Ann NY Acad Sci* 1993;696:216–26.

121 Turka LA, Dayton J, Sinclair G, Thompson CB, Mitchell BS. Guanine ribonucleotide depletion inhibits T cell activation. Mechanism of action of the immunosuppressive drug mizoribine. *J Clin Invest* 1991;87:940–8.

122 Griffith BP, Bando K, Hardesty RL *et al.* A prospective randomized trial of FK506 versus cyclosporine after human pulmonary transplantation. *Transplantation* 1994;57:848–51.

123 Keenan RJ, Konishi H, Kawai A *et al.* Clinical trial of tacrolimus versus cyclosporine in lung transplantation. *Ann Thorac Surg* 1995;60:580–5.

124 Paradis IL, Duncan SR, Dauber JH *et al.* Effect of augmented immunosuppression on human chronic lung allograft rejection. *Am Rev Respir Dis* 1992;145:A705.

125 Glanville AR, Bladwin J, Burke C, Theodore J, Robin ED. Obliterative bronchiolitis after heart-lung transplantation: apparent arrest by augmented immunosuppression. *Ann Intern Med* 1987;107:300–4.

126 Sollinger HW, Deierhoi MH, Belzer FO, Diethelm AG, Kauffman RS. RS-61443–a phase I clinical trial and pilot rescue study. *Transplantation* 1992;53:428–32.

127 Morris RE, Huang X, Gregory CR *et al.* Studies in experimental models of chronic rejection: use of rapamycin (sirolimus) and isoxazole derivatives (leflunomide and its analogue) for the suppression of graft vascular disease and obliterative bronchiolitis. *Transplant Proc* 1995;27:2068–9.

128 Bartlett RR, Dimitrijevic M, Mattar T *et al.* Leflunomide (HWA 486), a novel immunomodulating compound for the treatment of autoimmune disorders and reactions leading to transplantation rejection. *Agents Actions* 1991;32:10–21.

129 Takao M, Higenbottam TW, Audley T, Otulana BA, Wallwork J. Effects of inhaled nebulized steroids (Budesonide) on acute and chronic lung function in heart-lung transplant patients. *Transplant Proc* 1995;27:1284–5.

192

130 O'Riordan TG, Iacono A, Keenan RJ et al. Delivery and distribution of aerosolized cyclosporine in lung allograft recipients. Am J Respir Crit Care Med 1995;151:516–21.

131 Keenan RJ, Zeevi A, Iacono AT et al. Efficacy of inhaled cyclosporine in lung transplant recipients with refractory rejection: correlation of intragraft cytokine gene expression with pulmonary function and histologic characteristics. Surgery 1995;118:385–91.

132 Novick RJ, Schafers HJ, Stitt L et al. Seventy-two pulmonary retransplantations for obliterative bronchiolitis: predictors of survival. Ann Thorac Surg 1995;60:111–16.

133 Kirk AJ, Conacher ID, Corris PA, Ashcroft T, Dark JH. Successful surgical management of bronchial dehiscence after single-lung transplantation. Ann Thorac Surg 1990;49:147–9.

134 Schafers HJ, Schafer CM, Zink C, Haverich A, Borst HG. Surgical treatment of airway complications after lung transplantation. J Thorac Cardiovasc Surg 1994;107:1476–80.

135 Dumon JF. A dedicated tracheobronchial stent. Chest 1990;97:328–32.

136 Spatenka J, Khaghani A, Irving JD et al. Gianturco self-expanding metallic stents in treatment of tracheobronchial stenosis after single lung and heart and lung transplantation. Eur J Cardiothorac Surg 1991;5:648–52.

137 Klein E, Ernberg I, Masucci MG et al. T-cell response to B-cells and Epstein–Barr virus antigens in infectious mononucleosis. Cancer Res 1981;41:4210–15.

138 Armitage JM, Kormos RL, Stuart RS et al. Posttransplant lymphoproliferative disease in thoracic organ transplant patients: ten years of cyclosporine-based immunosuppresion. J Heart Lung Transplant 1991;10:877–86.

139 Garrett TJ, Chadburn A, Barr ML et al. Posttransplantation lymphoproliferative disorders treated with cyclophosphamide-doxorubicin-vincristine-prednisone chemotherapy. Cancer 1993;72:2782–5.

140 Fischer A, Blanche S, Le Bidois J et al. Anti-B-cell monoclonal antibodies in the treatment of severe B-cell lymphoproliferative syndrome following bone marrow and organ transplantation. N Engl J Med 1991;324:1451–56.

141 Faro A, Kurland G, Michaels MG et al. Interferon-alpha affects the immune response in post-transplant lymphoproliferative disorder. Am J Respir Crit Care Med 1996;153:1442–7.

142 Taguchi Y, Purtilo DT, Okano M. The effect of intravenous immunoglobulin and interferon-alpha on Epstein–Barr virus-induced lymphoproliferative disorder in a liver transplant recipient. Transplantation 1994;57:1813–15.

143 Lake KD. Management of drug interactions with cyclosporine. Pharmacotherapy 1991;11:110S–118S.

144 Schutz E, Gummert J, Mohr FW, Armstrong VW, Oellerich M. Azathioprine myelotoxicity related to elevated 6-thioguanine nucleotides in heart transplantation. Transplant Proc 1995;27:1298–300.

145 Read AE, Wiesner RH, LaBrecque DR et al. Hepatic veno-occlusive disease associated with renal transplantation and azathioprine therapy. Ann Intern Med 1986;104:651–5.

146 Rosenkranz HS, Klopman G. A re-examination of the genotoxicity and carcinogenicity of azathioprine. Mutat Res 1991;251:157–61.

147 Elsasser W, von Eickstedt KW. Corticotropins and corticosteroids. In: Dukes MNG. ed. Meyler's side effects of drugs, 12th edn. Amsterdam: Elsevier Science Publishers, 1992.

11 The current status of thoracic organ xenotransplantation

Peter C Braidley and John Wallwork

Xenotransplantation is the transplantation of tissues or organs from one species to another and shares a common origin with the concept of organ transplantation itself. The very first kidney transplants performed on patients with terminal uraemia by Jaboulay, Unger and others between 1906 and 1913 used kidneys from pigs, goats, and monkeys. Some initial function of the xenografts was reported but they inevitably failed within a short period of time. These experiments demonstrated that it was technically possible to implant and revascularise an organ which might, given optimal circumstances, then be expected to function. Interest then waned in the face of the poor results and it was not until the early 1960s that there was a resurgence of interest in xenotransplantation. Throughout the 1950s there had been significant improvements in the experimental and clinical results of allotransplantation with the introduction of new immuno-suppressive agents. However, with limited intensive care facilities and without the concept of brainstem death, the number and quality of cadaver organ donors was limited.

In an attempt to circumvent this problem Reemtsma and Starzl commenced clinical xenotransplant studies in 1963–1964. Reemtsma reported six patients who had chimpanzee renal xenografts with a maximum survival of nine months.[1] Episodes of acute rejection were successfully reversed in some cases.[2] Starzl reported six patients who had baboon renal xenografts with survivals of 10–49 days.[3] Ten out of 12 of these patients died of infectious complications due to the relatively crude immunosuppressive regime. In the intervening 30 years only about a dozen further xenografts have been attempted.

In contrast, over the same period of time allotransplantation has expanded dramatically with continuing improvements in outcome as judged by both quality of life and survival.[4,5] This has proved to be the Achilles heel of transplantation – with improving results the number of

194

patients being referred for transplant assessment has increased greatly and for many years now the demand for human organs has far outstripped supply. We have now come full circle and xenotransplantation is again being considered as one way of alleviating the donor organ shortage. A large body of experimental work with *in vitro* experiments and *in vivo* transplantation models has recently allowed a greater understanding of the processes involved in the rejection of xenograft organs. Concurrent advances in biotechnology have made it possible for these responses to be manipulated at a molecular level. This rapid growth in knowledge and the experimental successes seen so far suggest that xenotransplantation will soon be an effective clinical tool in the treatment of organ failure.

This chapter presents an up-to-date and coherent picture of the current status in human xenotransplantation. Necessarily, therefore, much of the detailed experimental background will be omitted and will instead be presented as a distillation of the different models studied to give an overall view. The emphasis of this chapter will also be on the most likely clinical scenario – that of pig-to-human xenotransplantation.

Past clinical experience of thoracic organ xenotransplantation

Dr James Hardy performed the first cardiac xenotransplant in January 1964 on a 68-year-old man with terminal heart failure in whom it had originally been planned to perform a human heart transplant.[70] His condition deteriorated rapidly and he was supported on cardiopulmonary bypass as his own heart failed but no suitable human donor was available. Instead, it was decided to perform a xenotransplant using the heart from a 43 kg chimpanzee. Surgical implantation was successful and the transplanted heart commenced beating forcefully but it soon became apparent that the undersized heart would not be able to support the patient's circulation and approximately one hour after discontinuing bypass, further support was withdrawn and the patient died.

Further attempts at clinical xenotransplantation were sporadic; in September 1967 the first lung xenotransplant was performed by Hitchcock and Haglin in Minneapolis. They transplanted the lung from a baboon into a patient who sadly died shortly afterwards. In 1968 Cooley[6] and Ross[7] made unsuccessful attempts to implant sheep and pig hearts respectively into patients with terminal heart failure.

Little was then reported until 1977 when Barnard performed two heterotopic cardiac xenotransplants as a method of providing left heart assistance in patients with cardiogenic shock after cardiopulmonary bypass.[8] The first patient was a 25-year-old female who had undergone aortic valve replacement and could not be weaned from cardiopulmonary bypass despite maximum conventional support. The heart of a 30 kg male baboon was transplanted heterotopically after which it was possible to discontinue all mechanical support. However, the patient suffered several episodes of ventricular fibrillation during which time the baboon heart alone was unable to support the circulation. Six hours after completion of the transplant, the baboon heart also went into ventricular fibrillation and all attempts at resuscitation were unsuccessful. Histological evaluation of the transplanted heart revealed no evidence of rejection. A second patient with poor ventricular function received heterotopic assistance from the heart of a chimpanzee, also after aortic valve replacement. This patient survived for four days before the native heart ceased functioning and again the smaller heterotopic heart was unable to support the circulation. Histological evaluation of the chimpanzee heart showed severe rejection, despite treating the recipient with conventional immunosuppression.

Of all the clinical attempts at xenotransplantation, perhaps the most attention was elicited by the "Baby Fae" case.[9] She was diagnosed as having the hypoplastic left heart syndrome shortly after birth and after discussion with her family, on 26 October 1984 she underwent orthotopic heart xenotransplantation with a heart obtained from a size-matched but ABO-incompatible baboon. Immunosuppression was with cyclosporin A alone and good progress was made for the first 11 days, at which time she was treated with a bolus of methylprednisolone for presumed rejection. By day 14 elevated creatine kinase levels and echocardiography indicated impairment of xenograft function and further methylprednisolone was administered. She continued to deteriorate and by day 17 was reintubated, ventilated, and treated with additional antirejection therapy of antithymocyte globulin and azathioprine. In spite of this additional therapy, the function of the heart xenograft continued to deteriorate and she died 20 days after her xenotransplant. The xenograft showed only traces of a cell-mediated response but features of humorally mediated injury were more marked. Xenograft failure appeared to be due to progressive antibody-mediated mechanisms that were not modified by the immunosuppressive regime used.

The most recent thoracic xenotransplant was performed in 1992 by a group in Poland who transplanted a pig heart into a patient with Marfan's disease.[10] At operation the patient was put on cardiopulmonary bypass and the patient's blood was first perfused through two pig hearts. A third heart was then transplanted orthotopically and the patient was successfully weaned from cardiopulmonary bypass. For the first four hours his condition was stable but thereafter his condition deteriorated and a low cardiac output syndrome developed which it was not possible to reverse. The patient died 23 h postoperatively.

Why consider xenotransplantation?

The primary motive for the resurgence of interest in xenotransplantation is seeking a way to meet the demand for transplantation which cannot currently be met because of a shortage of organ donors. The number of organ donors in the United Kingdom has remained relatively constant in recent years and even if all the potential donor organs could be retrieved, this would still be inadequate to meet current demands.[11] Figure 11.1a illustrates the situation for renal transplantation with an ever-widening gap between the number of kidney transplants performed and the number of patients on the waiting list. A similar graph plotted for thoracic organ transplantation (Figure 11.1b) shows no significant increase in the number of transplants performed since 1989. In the absence of any widely available supportive treatment for these patients, there is a high mortality rate whilst waiting for a transplant: up to 30% of patients at our hospital will die before a suitable donor organ becomes available.

The use of animals as donors for human transplantation is an attractive possibility because current demands could easily be met and the indications and stringent selection criteria for transplantation could be reevaluated to offer this form of treatment to a wider cohort of patients. The transplant could be performed as an elective procedure to occur at an optimal time for the individual patient. This would greatly reduce the need for operating overnight, as usually occurs at present, and would therefore allow better planning and use of resources. The ability to identify a donor for any recipient well before a transplant took place could allow specific intervention in that donor – recipient combination to further facilitate successful engraftment; for example, the induction of T and/or B cell tolerance.

Potential donor species

The first working classification of xenograft combinations was made by Sir Roy Calne in 1969.[12] In this original definition xenografts were divided into "concordant" and "discordant" categories based upon the temporal nature of the rejection process. Those in which rejection occurred over a period of a few days, analogous to allograft rejection, were termed "concordant". In contrast, those which were rejected hyperacutely within minutes or hours, as occurred in sensitised recipients of allografts, were termed "discordant". The "concordant" xenografts were observed to be between species that were quite closely related phylogenetically, for example baboon to human, whereas those xenografts described as "discordant" were between phylogenetically more distant species, for example pig to human. In experimental models of xenotransplantation using "concordant" combinations, it has been possible to achieve long-term xenograft survival with relatively simple immunosuppressive protocols.

(a)

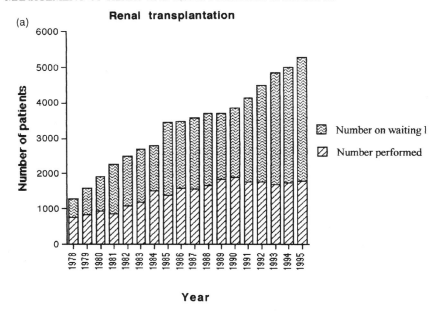

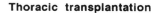

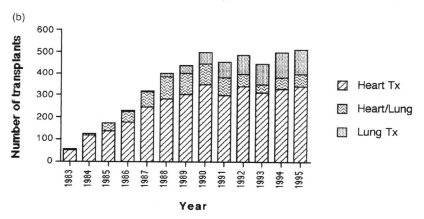

Fig 11.1 (a) The increasing gap between supply of organs and demand for transplantation as demonstrated in renal transplantation. (b) The initial increase in number of thoracic transplants performed but with a finite donor organ supply numbers have remained essentially constant since 1989 (data supplied by UK Transplant Support Service Agency).

198

Table 11.1   Reported cases of thoracic zenotransplantation with both concordant and discordant donor animals

Year	Organ	Donor	Survival	Notes	
1964	Heart	Chimpanzee	1 h	Hardy[70]	Orthotopic
1967	Lung	Baboon	Hours	Hitchcock	Orthotopic
1968	Heart	Sheep	Hours	Cooley[6]	Orthotopic
1968	Heart	Pig	Hours	Ross[7]	Orthotopic
1977	Heart	Baboon	6 h	Barnard[8]	Heterotopic
1977	Heart	Baboon	4 days	Barnard[8]	Heterotopic
1985	Heart	Baboon	20 days	Bailey[9]	Orthotopic
1992	Heart	Pig	24 h	Czaplicki[10]	Orthotopic

However, this has not been the case until very recently for "discordant" combinations because of the difficulty in overcoming hyperacute rejection.

Most of the previous clinical experience of xenotransplantation has been using "concordant" primate donors – either chimpanzees or baboons. Although this may have been considered preferential in that the rejection process was less vigorous, there are other significant drawbacks that mean these animals may only be used in limited situations. Instead, attention has recently focused upon the domestic pig as being the most likely donor animal for human xenotransplantation.[13] Although this animal represents a "discordant" species, it has recently been demonstrated that it is possible to avoid hyperacute rejection through genetic manipulation of the donor pig (see below) thus converting it into a functionally "concordant" species. Having thus removed the main immunological advantage of primates as donors, the pig has many other advantages.

Xenotransplantation aims to remove the restriction caused by limited donor availability and so donor animals have to be available in sufficient numbers to meet the projected demand for organs. Pigs breed easily in captivity, have large litters, and grow rapidly to full adult size, thus ensuring that supply can far exceed demand. On the other hand, primates are far more difficult to breed, have low parity, and develop only slowly. The transplanted organs must be capable of adequate function to maintain the recipient and so must be comparable in terms of physiology and, importantly, size. Clinical experience in thoracic transplantation of both allografts and xenografts demonstrates that organs too small for the recipient will fail. Few primates in captivity reach even 40–50 kg but pigs can easily be available in an appropriate size to match even the largest human recipient.

The potential risk of disease transmission from donor animal to human recipient has to be considered. Both pigs and primates carry zoonotic organisms that may be transmitted to man, of particular concern being the transmission of potentially lethal simian viruses, only some of which can be identified. To reduce this risk, pigs are being raised in specific pathogen-free conditions designed to minimise the potential for infection occurring in the donor herd. Ongoing microbiological surveillance will identify any individual animals with potential pathogens. These can then be removed from the herd and culled.

Pathophysiology of xenograft rejection

Hyperacute rejection

The process of hyperacute rejection (HXR) leads to the rapid and inevitable loss of graft function within a few minutes or hours of revascularisation. Several models have been studied to help understand the mechanisms involved but most of the data have been obtained in the pig-to-human combination. This has been achieved by using an *ex vivo* working heart model perfusing pig hearts with human blood and *in vivo* experiments observing the interaction of pig endothelial cells with human blood components. Data can also be extrapolated from *in vivo* transplantation experiments using non-human primate recipients.

This process evolves at the endothelial cell-blood interface as soon as the xenograft is revascularised. It involves preformed xenoreactive antibodies binding to specific epitopes on the endothelial cell surface of the xenograft with the consequent activation of both the complement cascade and the endothelium itself. This in turn sets up a train of events damaging the endothelial cells and promoting intravascular coagulation, leading to rapid organ failure. The roles and interactions of these components will now be discussed in greater detail.

Histopathology

The pathological features of organs hyperacutely rejected are easily recognisable and careful histological analysis gives valuable insight into the mechanisms involved. Paraffin sections stained with haematoxylin and eosin show widespread haemorrhage and oedema causing massive disruption of the normal architecture. Many of the vessels in the xenografts show endothelial cell necrosis and are occluded with platelet and fibrin thrombi. Any cellular infiltrate into these organs is usually scanty and consists of polymorphs and mononuclear cells. Immunohistochemical analysis shows deposition on the vascular endothelium of antibody, predominantly IgM but also some IgG, along with components of the complement system, importantly C1q, C3, C4, and C9. Fibrinogen is also seen, as are markers of endothelial cell activation – TNFα, IFNγ, E-selectin, tissue factor, and ICAM-1.

Target antigens in hyperactive rejection

The binding of xenoreactive antibodies to their appropriate ligands on vascular endothelium initiates the process of HXR. These target antigens have been found to be glycoproteins in the 115–135 kD range with the specific target antigen being located on the carbohydrate moiety rather than the polypeptide determinants. Human xenoreactive antibodies recognise targets containing immunodominant galactosyl residues located on complex N-linked oligosaccarides.[14] This target is a linear-B carbohydrate structure containing a Gal(α1-3)Gal linkage that has become known as the αGal epitope.[15]

The presence of this α-galactosyl epitope is generated by the enzyme α1-3 galactosyl transferase (α1,3GT) which transfers a terminal galactose residue to a subterminal galactose on glycoproteins and glycolipids within the Golgi apparatus. This enzyme is found to be active in non-primate mammals, prosimians, and New World monkeys but is absent in Old World monkeys, apes, and humans.[16] The α1,3GT gene has been cloned from cow and mouse cDNA libraries and these have been used to identify a homologous gene in humans. This, however, contains nonsense and frameshift mutations rendering the gene a non-functional pseudogene.[17] Comparative sequencing of this gene in primates suggests it was inactivated after the divergence of apes from monkeys some 28 million years ago. One possible mechanism for this is that evolutionary selection pressure brought about the inactivation of the α1,3GT gene. An infectious agent detrimental to primates which expressed α-galactosyl or related epitopes may have brought about deletion of the gene, allowing the subsequent production of anti-αGal antibodies as a means of defence.[18] The Gal(α1-3)Gal epitope is the main structure on pig tissues recognised by human xenoreactive antibodies and is present in a number of related carbohydrates. There appear to be at least five major molecules which carry this epitope and others that carry it in lesser amounts. All of these are important in a passive role as sites for the binding of antibody and complement. Some may also have active roles in endothelial cell activation but this remains to be elucidated.

Preformed xenoreactive antibodies

Xenoreactive antibodies belong to the group termed "natural antibodies" which arise without prior exposure to their target antigen. They are polyreactive and bind with low avidity to a large number of self and exogenous antigens. These antibodies are present in relatively large amounts and are predominantly of the IgM class and can be demonstrated to be polyreactive by the ability of ssDNA and thyroglobulin to inhibit binding to xenogeneic antigens in an inhibition ELISA. The titre of human xenoreactive IgM antibodies against pig aortic endothelial cells has been found to vary considerably between individuals (up to 400-fold) and they represent around 0.1% of the total IgM in the sera tested.[19] There are also IgG xenoreactive antibodies, in particular the anti-αGal antibody, a polyclonal natural antibody which interacts specifically with the α-

galactosyl epitope and constitutes around 1% of all circulating IgG.[20] In common with the blood group antibodies, it is likely that anti-Gal results from constant stimulation by enterobacteria of bacterial lipopolysaccharides that express the α-galactosyl epitope on their outer membranes.[21] The titre of anti-Gal antibodies also varies considerably between individuals and the degree of cytotoxicity of human serum to pig kidney cells correlates with the titre of anti-αGal antibodies.[22]

The precise role of polyreactive antibodies remains unclear though they probably play an important part in the initial defence of self against invading microorganisms. They are thought to derive from a CD5+ population of B lymphocytes and in the immunologically naive infant, these represent the majority of B lymphocytes in cord blood.[23] The frequency and polyreactive nature of these CD5+ lymphocytes suggest they would provide most of the precursors of the antibody-producing cells in the primary response to any defined antigen, though the low affinity of these antibodies may preclude complete clearance. High-affinity monospecific IgG antibodies produced later may achieve this but whether any of the clones of CD5+ cells involved in the primary response give rise to cells producing specific antibodies is unclear. The origin of these polyreactive antibodies is phylogenetically ancient and represents an early stage in the development of an effective immune system and they are the only antibodies found in primitive creatures such as the shark or torpedo fish.[24]

Complement

The activation of complement plays a pivotal role in the hyperacute rejection of xenografts. Complement deposition can be demonstrated on the endothelium of rejected organs by immunohistochemistry and can be shown to be depleted from the recipient serum over the period of time in which rejection occurs. If complement is inactivated[25,26] or if complement deficient animal models are used[27] then hyperacute rejection can be avoided and survival prolonged.

The activation of the complement cascade is shown in Figure 11.2 and can be initiated through two different pathways. In the classic pathway, antibody is required to bind the complement component C1q and so activate the C1 complex, triggering the rest of the cascade. Activation via the alternative pathway is independent of antibody and occurs through the spontaneous hydrolysis of C3 with the generation of C3b and ultimately the alternative pathway C3 convertase C3bBb. This pathway can be seen to act as a positive feedback loop for the classic pathway with generation of increasing amounts of C3b, as well as acting independently. The alternative pathway has been identified in two experimental models as the cause of hyperacute rejection in the absence of xenoreactive antibody.[28,29]

Complement activation has a number of important effects that contribute to hyperacute rejection. The membrane attack complex inserts into the cell membrane and contributes to cell lysis by disturbing the normal resting cell membrane potential and the fluxes of Na^+, K^+, and Ca^{++}. The anaphylatoxins C3a and C5a are potent proinflammatory mediators. Both cause histamine release from mast cells and basophils, contraction of smooth muscle, and increased permeability of vessels. Additionally, C5a activates endothelial cells[30] and is a powerful chemoattractant for granulocytes and monocytes. Activation of these cells through their C5a receptor causes lysosomal enzyme release and the production of reactive oxygen species by neutrophils and the synthesis and release of cytokines by

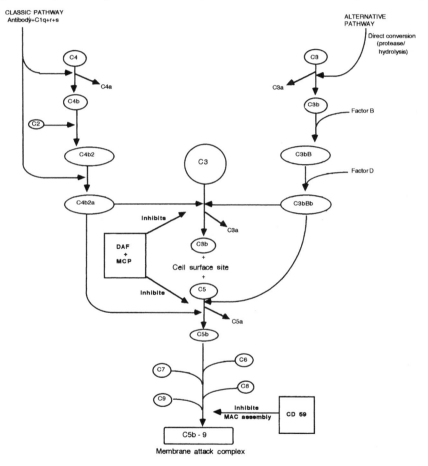

Fig 11.2 Complement activation. The complement activation pathways. The regulators of complement activation DAF, MCP, and CD59 are shown at their site of action. DAF, decay-accelerating factor; MCP, membrane cofactor protein; CD 59.

monocytes. Neutrophil adherence to the endothelium is promoted by the upregulation of complement receptors 1 and 3 and by the endothelial deposition of iC3b that serves as an accessory adhesion molecule for cells expressing CR1 and CR3.[31]

The endothelium

The interface between vascular endothelium and blood is the first site of interaction between the donor and recipient. In the normal situation the resting, quiescent endothelium promotes a local environment that prevents the generation of thrombin and the adherence of leucocytes. It also maintains a tight physical barrier that prevents leakage of the contents of the vascular space into the parenchyma and vice-versa. However, this situation can easily change and it has been shown *in vitro* that endothelial cells exposed to certain stimuli undergo metabolic and structural changes and become "activated".[32] These changes lead to a local environment that is procoagulant, enabling fibrin generation, neutrophil adhesion, and margination to occur. Many of these changes are seen in organs undergoing hyperacute rejection, suggesting that endothelial cell activation is also an important component in this process. The precise mechanism of endothelial cell activation has not been clearly defined but the involvement of antibody and complement is essential. *In vitro*, the addition of antibody alone to cultured porcine endothelial cells will cause some degree of activation[33] but antibody and complement together act synergistically to cause a far greater degree of activation.[34]

The events of endothelial cell activation have been conceptually divided into two categories: type 1 activation (or stimulation) which occurs rapidly and does not require *de novo* protein synthesis; and type 2 activation which develops slowly over hours or days and requires gene expression or suppression.[35] Some of the target antigens on the surface of porcine endothelial cells resemble human integrins[36] and this finding may help provide a mechanism for some of the events seen in both type 1 and 2 activation.

The continuity of the endothelial cell monolayer is in part maintained by integrin $\alpha_2\beta_1$ complexes and binding of antibody to either of these chains will cause the development of "holes", so compromising the integrity of the monolayer.[37] When porcine endothelial cells are incubated with human serum, phase-contrast microscopy can demonstrate the appearance of intercellular gaps or pores. This response is dependent upon the presence of antibody and C5b-7 but not C8 or C9.[38] Retraction and "pore formation" of the otherwise confluent endothelial cell layer will result in an increased fluid flux across the vessel wall, so leading to interstitial oedema. Retraction of this layer will expose the subendothelial matrix containing collagen and tissue factor which will trigger platelet adhesion and activation of the extrinsic pathway of coagulation. A process of regulated exocytosis leads to the elaboration of stored substances including prostacyclin, platelet-activating factor, and tissue factor, along with the translocation of P-selectin to the endothelial cell surface. These act further to promote platelet and neutrophil adhesion and activation. The prothrombotic environment is further enhanced by the loss of heparan sulphate from the cell surface. The glycosaminoglycan branches of this molecule bind circulating antithrombin III to produce a powerful antithrombotic effect by inhibiting the generation of thrombin. It also anchors the enzyme superoxide dismutase which acts to reduce oxidant-mediated damage.

Delayed Xenograft Rejection

Organs transplanted between "concordant" combinations or between "discordant" combinations in which hyperacute rejection is prevented are found to reject in an accelerated fashion over a period of days. The histopathological features and kinetics of this process suggest that it is neither classic hyperacute rejection nor a rapid form of a first-set allograft rejection. A spectrum of histological changes is observed with elements of both cellular and humoral rejection being present though the precise pattern observed depends upon the particular animal model studied. In a few *very* closely related species a predominantly cellular pattern of xenograft rejection is seen but if there is any significant phylogenetic difference between the two species, a vigorous form of humoral rejection known as delayed xenograft rejection (DXR) is observed. It is clear that understanding of this rejection process is vital if long-term xenograft survival is to be achieved.

Histopathology

The histopathological features of DXR in heart xenografts are characterised by gradually increasing myocytolysis with loss of myofilaments and disruption of architectural continuity. Some interstitial oedema and haemorrhage may also be seen. Vascular changes are evident with perivascular space with leucocytes occurs and ultimately thrombosis of some vessels is seen. In comparison to allograft rejection, the degree of perivascular and interstitial infiltration with monocytes and lymphocytes is less. Immunohistochemical analysis of these rejected xenografts reveals endothelial deposition of immunoglobulin, mainly IgM though some IgG can also be seen, along the co-deposition of components of the classic pathway of complement activation.

The role of antibody

The importance of antibody in DXR has only quite recently been fully appreciated. It had been thought that concordant xenograft rejection represented a vigorous form of cellular rejection given the similarities in the timescale of rejection and the observation that in a few models survival matched or even exceeded allograft survival.[39] However, long-term survival proved elusive despite immunosuppressive strategies that were successful in allografts. The importance of antibody as the primary effector of rejection in these models was first acknowledged after two sets of experiments. Nude rats have no T cells and can thus accept allografts indefinitely without the need for immunosuppression. However, when these rats were transplanted with hamster hearts it was found that they rejected at the same pace and with the same histological features as in normal T cell-component rats.[40,41] Similarly, if normal rats are treated with large doses of monoclonal antibodies to eliminate the T cell repertoire, survival of hamster heart xenografts is not prolonged.[42] When serum from these recipients is analysed, a significant rise in the titre of antidonor antibodies can be seen at the time of rejection. The kinetics of this response are such that a rise in the serum titre is not seen until the second day posttransplantation with a peak at around five days and, when put through a fractionation column, reveals predominantly an IgM response. Passive transfer experiments using this fraction will lead to the hyperacute rejection of hamster hearts in rat recipients. The specificity of these antibodies is not yet clear – they are not donor specific but are species specific as they will react with cells from a different hamster strain so it is unlikely that donor MHC is a specific target. The target antigens are T cell-independent antigens as T cell help is not required for antibody production.

Complement

As well as its role in hyperacute rejection, complement can be shown to play a role in DXR. As may be expected, a rise in antidonor antibody titres will lead to classic pathway complement activation. Depletion of complement alone in rat recipients of hamster hearts will prolong survival by a few days. When combined with Cyclosporin A for effective cellular immunosuppression, survival is further prolonged though a significant rise in the titre of antidonor antibodies is still seen by the time of rejection.[44] Depletion of complement may be effective as "rescue therapy" in acute xenograft rejection associated with sudden rises in antidonor antibody titres.

Cell-mediated xenograft rejection

The cell-mediated response to a xenograft will have to be controlled once hyperacute rejection and the subsequent induced humoral response have overcome. There is as yet no common consensus as to the importance and strength of the cellular response to xenogeneic organs. Interpretation of the available data is often confusing because many different species combinations have been studied and conflicting results have been obtained within the same species combinations.

In the primary allogeneic response, donor MHC antigens can be recognised directly by recipient T cells without the need for their peptides to be processed and presented with self MHC molecules (direct presentation). It has been suggested that xenogeneic MHC antigens do not sufficiently resemble self MHC molecules and accordingly cannot be recognised as intact molecules by recipient T cell receptors. Instead, they have first to be processed by antigen-presenting cells and are then subsequently presented in association with recipient class II MHC molecules (indirect presentation). There are also suggestions that some of the other molecular interactions important in T cell activation, for example interactions with CD8 molecules, adhesion molecules, and costimulatory cytokines, might be defective in the xenogeneic situation due to molecular incompatibilities between species. Initial studies showed a much weaker primary response *in vitro* when mouse T cells were cultured with primate or pig stimulator cells than was seen with allogeneic mouse stimulator cells.[45] *In vivo* experiments using mice recipients depleted of CD4+ cells showed that xenogeneic skin grafts survived longer than allogeneic skin grafts on the same recipients.[46] These data (and others) were held to indicate that cell-mediated rejection might be weaker in xenogeneic combinations than in an allogeneic system.

More recent experiments have brought this hypothesis into question. "Knock-out" mice have recently become available that are deficient in mouse MHC antigens. Transplantation studies have shown that allogeneic donor organs that lack MHC to stimulate recipient T cells directly are still rejected rapidly by sensitisation through the indirect pathway. Subsequently xenogeneic skin graft rejection by sensitisation through the indirect pathway. Subsequently xenogeneic skin graft rejection has been studied in mice that lack class II MHC antigens but have normal CD4+ counts. These mice still rapidly rejected pig skin grafts but not if the CD4+ cells were depleted. This again suggests the importance of the CD4+ cell in xenograft cell-mediated rejection but through a direct stimulation pathway by donor APCs as the class II MHC necessary for indirect presentation are absent. This is contrary to the *in vivo* data suggesting there was no direct stimulation. It has also been suggested that the xenogeneic cell-mediated response might be stronger than the allogeneic response from experiments using mice in which the survival of allogeneic but not xenogeneic skin grafts could be prolonged by high doses of cyclosporin A. Similarly, mice which have a defect of their CD3 molecule leading to virtually no T cell activation will reject xenogeneic skin grafts within a few weeks but allogeneic skin grafts are indefinitely accepted.[47]

It is difficult to draw any conclusions as to the strength and nature of the human antipig cell-mediated response although *in vitro* experiments have suggested that there are both strong direct and indirect responses by human T cells to porcine stimulating cells[48] and it is likely that CD4+ lymphocytes play an important role. Attention will have to be paid to the possibility of unusual cytokine responses, the failure of normal inhibitors of inflammation to work across species barriers, and the role of non T cell-mediated cell killing, possibly by NK cells.

Current strategies to prevent xenograft rejection

Hyperacute rejection

This is the first and perhaps the most difficult obstacle to overcome in seeking to achieve successful long-term discordant xenograft survival and attention has focused upon the removal of xenoreactive antibodies and the inhibition of complement activity to try and prolong survival.

Antibody depletion

Depletion of xenoreactive antibodies in the recipient has been achieved by organ perfusion or by plasmapheresis and these techniques have been shown to prolong survival by several days.[49-51] The depletion of antibody titres is only transient and a rebound phenomenon is often seen. Organ perfusion may additionally sensitise the recipient with the development of high titres of antiendothelial IgM and IgG antibodies. A more useful application of this approach would be using immunoaffinity columns containing α1-3Gal ligands that would absorb out human xenoreactive antibodies as blood passed through the column. This might be used as an adjunct to other measures just prior to implantation or as rescue in the event of a later rise in antidonor antibody titres.

Complement inhibition

As outlined earlier in this chapter, activation of the complement cascade is central to the process of HXR. The control and inhibition of this pathway is considered by many workers in the field of xenotransplantation to be the key to overcoming hyperacute rejection and achieving successful long-term xenograft survival.

Pharmacological inhibition of complement was first achieved using cobra venom factor which rapidly depletes recipient C3 and thus inactivates the complement system until sufficient C3 has been synthesised *de novo*. When used alone, it has been shown to prolong the survival of pig heart xenografts in primates from a few hours to several days and concurrent administration with other immunosuppressive agents has achieved survival of up to 25 days (DKC Cooper, personal communication). It has, however, to be administered parenterally on a regular basis and may be associated with problems of toxicity.

A more subtle approach being developed by several groups hinges upon the mechanisms by which complement activation is controlled in the normal individual (see below).

Delayed xenograft rejection

Most of the experimental work in preventing DXR has been done in rodent xenograft models and the strategies developed with them are being extrapolated for use in pig-to-primate xenograft models. Conventional immunosuppression with either cyclosporin A or FK 506 as monotherapy has been shown to be inadequate, prolonging survival by only a few days. It is clear that the induced antibody response to the donor organ has to be effectively suppressed for prolonged survival to be achieved. To prevent antibody production the rapid clonal expansion of xenoreactive B cells has to be prevented and consequently most of the agents used have been antimetabolites or inhibitors of DNA synthesis. The most effective agents used include cyclophosphamide, methotrexate, brequinar sodium, mycophenolate mofetil, and leflunamide. When used alone they produced considerably longer xenograft survival but rejection still ensued. Combination of these agents with either cyclosporin A or FK 506 produced further improvements with indefinite survival being achieved in a significant number of cases.[52,53]

The difficulty lies in extrapolating from these experiments into primate or human recipients of pig organs. There are undoubtedly going to be differences in the relative strengths of the immune response between species and also idiosyncratic differences in the degree of toxicity to the drugs used in the recipients. A combination of drugs may be needed to see a useful effect whilst minimising drug toxicity.

Regulation of complement activation

Complement is a cascade system that can deliver a rapid and amplified response following activation at only a few sites. Under normal conditions there is some degree of continuous activation which needs to be down regulated to prevent otherwise uncontrolled activation which would damage the individual's own cells. This is achieved through the action of a number of fluid–phase and membrane-bound proteins known as regulators of complement activation (RCAs). Particular attention has been paid to complement receptor type 1 (CR1), decay-accelerating factor (DAF), and membrane cofactor protein (MCP) which act to inhibit the C3/C5 convertases and CD59 which inhibits assembly of the membrane attack complex C5b-9 (MAC).

Complement receptor type 1

This is found chiefly on erythrocytes and functions to clear immune complexes via the liver by binding C3B and C4B. A soluble form of the human protein (sCR1) has been produced which lacks the transmembrane region but otherwise retains all the known functions of the membrane-bound form and is a powerful inhibitor of both pathways of complement activation. It binds to the C3b and C4b components of the C3/C5 convertase, thus preventing the generation of the inflammatory anaphyla-toxins C3a and C5a and assembly of the MAC. It also acts as a cofactor in the factor I-mediated degradation of C3b and C4b.

sCR1 will function across species barriers and was initially demonstrated to prolong xenograft survival in a guinea-pig to rat model in a dose-dependent manner.[54] It has subsequently been tested in a pig-to-cynomolgus monkey model with a single bolus dose prolonging heterotopic heart survival from $0.8 +/- 0.2$ h to $70 +/- 18$ h.[55] A con-tinuous infusion of sCR1 in the same model further prolonged survival to seven days before rejection occurred and further treatment with cyclosporin A and cyclophosphamide prolonged survival to 32 and 21 days in two cases (3rd International Congress on Xenotransplantation, Boston, 1995. Abstract #215).

Decay-accelerating factor, membrane cofactor protein and CD59

These molecules have a wider tissue distribution than CR1. DAF inhibits the formation of the classic and alternative pathway convertases and also accelerates their decay (Figure 11.3) MCP binds C3b and C4b and

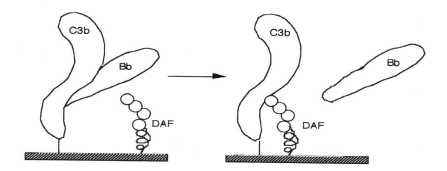

Fig 11.3 The decay-accelerating activity of DAF. DAF competes with the activation product of factor B (Bb) for a binding site on C3b and so inhibits the formation of a part of the C3/C5 convertases. It also competes with C2b for a site on C4b; thus, it can inhibit both the classic and alternative pathway convertases.

facilitates their cleavage by factor I, thus also inhibiting the function of the C3/C5 convertases. CD59, on the other hand, works by binding C8 and C9 to prevent formation of MAC. These proteins are all extremely efficient at downregulating the inappropriate activation of complement from their *own* species – a property known as "species restriction".[56] Thus, although pig organs may have effective RCAs against their own complement, these proteins would be unable to inhibit the activation of human complement, thus facilitating hyperacute rejection.

This understanding has provided the rationale for the approach adopted by several groups worldwide in seeking to produce pigs that could be used for human transplantation. If pigs were to express human RCAs on their cell surface it might be expected that they could downregulate human complement activation and thus HXR could be prevented. This hypothesis was first tested *in vitro* by transfecting mouse fibroblasts and porcine endothelial cells with cDNA for human DAF, MCP, and CD59. Once these transfected cell lines were established and found to express human proteins, they were exposed to human serum. Naive endothelial cells or fibroblasts were lysed in significant numbers by human serum whereas the transfected cells were protected from lysis by the human serum.[57,58] This evidence provides encouraging support for the hypotheses that if pig organs were to express functional human RCAs, they might be protected from HXR.

Transgenic technology

To create a pig that will express functional human RCAs on its cell surface, it is necessary to incorporate the human genes coding for those proteins into the genome of the pig itself, thus creating a transgenic pig. This newly inserted piece of genetic material has to be in a form and location that will allow transcription into mRNA and thence translation into protein before being expressed on the cell surface in a functional form. This is a complex process with the potential for failure at many levels.

Two different approaches have been used by the groups currently involved in this work. One approach has been to attach the genes for DAF and CD59 to specific human α- and β-globin promoters to achieve expression of DAF and CD59 on the surface of erythrocytes. Proteins expressed in this way will translocate from the erythrocyte cell membrane to the cell membranes of donor endothelial cells. Using this technique, prolonged survival (up to 30 h) of transgenic pig hearts transplanted heterotopically into baboons was seen, though no contemporaneous control results were reported.[59] The drawback of this approach would seem to be that the translocated RCA molecules will only have a limited duration on the cell surface and are not constitutively expressed.

The approach adopted by ourselves and others, in contrast, does lead to constitutive expression of these RCA molecules. We have used a 6.5 kb mini-gene construct for human DAF (hDAF) as the whole-gene construct was too large to be used with the available technology. This was first tested successfully in mice, with transgenic offspring being produced that had widespread expression of hDAF.[60] The technique was then translated to use in the pig. Fertilised ova are harvested from a donor pig and those at the single cell pronuclear zygote stage selected. Two thousand copies of the hDAF mini-gene are then injected into the pronucleus using microinjection techniques and the manipulated ova are then reimplanted into a surrogate mother whose oestrus is synchronous with the donor pig. There is then a wait of nearly four months whilst gestation occurs.

This process of incorporation into the pig genome is entirely random and depends upon spontaneously occurring breaks in the pig chromosomes. When this occurs the human DNA can insert itself into these breaks as the pig chromosome is being repaired. One or more copies may insert together on the same chromosome or integration may occur in two or more different chromosomes. In many cases integration does not occur at all. Our results have been quite encouraging given this rather random process. Around 2500 zygotes were microinjected and transferred to 85 pigs, of whom 49 delivered litters with 311 piglets being born. Of these, 49 were found to be transgenic with between one and 30 copies of the gene being incorporated.[61] These are all heterozygous for the hDAF gene and it is necessary to back-cross these and other generations to produce homozygous lines.

Expression of the transgene

The mere presence of the transgene in the pig genome is of little consequence unless it is producing a functional product. We have found that 33 out of 49 transgenic pigs produced mRNA for hDAF. Some of these were later sacrificed and their tissues examined for mRNA and hDAF. These studies have shown that hDAF is expressed on the cell surface of most of the organs tested and, in common with mRNA, the amount of expression varies from pig to pig and within different tissues from the same pig. Immunohistochemical staining for hDAF has confirmed its presence on the endothelium of the organs tested.[62]

This variability of expression is not unexpected given the random nature of the process. The control of gene expression is complex and for each gene there is a locus control region that regulates the level of gene transcption and therefore the level of protein expression. The mini-gene used does not include the appropriate locus control region and is therefore under the control of that region which regulates the pig DNA where the human DNA has incorporated. The level of expression is therefore integration site dependent. To try and overcome this problem, yeast artificial chromosome (YAC) technology is being investigated. Much larger genetic constructs can be carried into cells, thus allowing full genomic constructs to be used. This will allow all the different isoforms of the gene to be produced and appropriate locus control of the gene can be achieved, giving greater reproducibility of hDAF expression.

Functional assessment

The protective effect of hDAF has been tested in a number of *in vitro* models. Pig peripheral blood monocytes that expressed hDAF were protected from lysis by human complement when compared to normal pig monocytes.[63] Endothelial cell lines expressing hDAF obtained from culture of transgenic pig aortic endothelial cells have been studied. In a number of lines levels of expression of hDAF equal to or greater than human endothelial cell lines have been demonstrated.[64] These cell lines have also been shown to be protected from lysis by human complement.

An *ex vivo* working heart perfusion model has been used to study normal and transgenic pig heart. In this model, hearts are mounted on an artificial circulation apparatus so that the left ventricle has to pump blood around the circuit against a physiological afterload. This allows the manipulation and measurement of many different parameters. When normal pig hearts are perfused with human blood the cardiac output rapidly declines with a median survival time of 47 min. In contrast, hearts from transgenic pigs were found to have a much greater cardiac output and a much prolonged survival time of >240 min (Figure 11.4). Histological analysis of the transgenic pig hearts showed no evidence of complement deposition and much less damage than is seen in the normal pig hearts which show significant complement deposition.

Because of limitations in the *ex vivo* model further studies have been carried out using an *in vivo* transplant model. Hearts from normal control pigs and transgenic pigs have been transplanted heterotopically into untreated primate recipients (Figure 11.5). Hearts from normal pigs have a median survival of 1.6 days whereas the hearts from transgenic pigs have a significantly prolonged survival of 5.1 days (p<0.0001). A group of recipients were then immunosuppressed using cyclosporin A, cyclophosphamide, and methylprednisolone, five of whom received normal pig hearts and 10 of whom received transgenic pig hearts. In this imunosuppressed group, the median survival of normal pig hearts was 55 min and the median survival of transgenic hearts was 40 days (p<0.0001). The majority of the recipients of transgenic pig hearts were sacrificed with beating hearts in line with Home Office animal welfare guidelines because of systemic complications of diarrhoea and anaemia. Histological examination of these hearts showed no cellular infiltrate or any other evidence of immune-mediated damage.[65]

Future approaches

The results obtained so far are extremely encouraging and serve to stimulate research into areas that may further improve the outcome of pig organ xenografts. Improvements in complement down regulation may be achieved by the use of multiple constructs for different RCAs within the same animal and use of YAC constructs may allow the use of full genomic DNA with locus control to facilitate optimal expression of the transgene in all tissues.

Attention is being directed to the gal(α1-3)gal sugar present on the surface of porcine endothelial cells that is the prime target epitope of human xenoreactive antibodies. This epitope could be masked by the

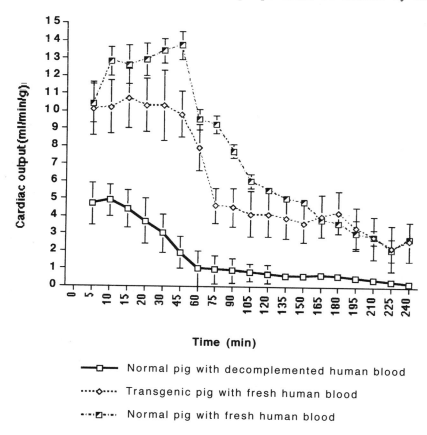

Fig 11.4   Cardiac function of pig hearts perfused with human blood. It can be seen that normal pig hearts have poor initial function and deteriorate quickly whereas the transgenic pig hearts or normal pig hearts perfused with decomplemented human blood have much greater initial function and decline less rapidly.

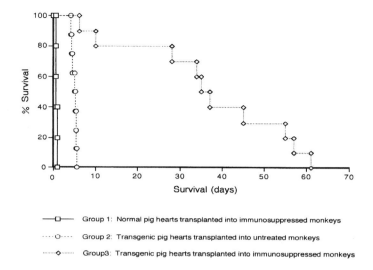

Fig 11.5   Transgenic pig heart survival. This graph shows the survival of normal and transgenic pig hearts when transplanted heterotopically into the abdomen of cynomolgus monkeys. Treatment with cyclosporin A, cyclophosphamide, and steroids prolongs survival to a median of 40 days.

addition of sialic acid to the epitope using current transgenic technology to pigs transgenic for the enzyme sialyl transferase. The modified epitope would then be masked from human xenoreactive antibodies. Germline deletion of the gene coding for the enzyme by homologous restriction to produce a "knock-out" pig that lacked the enzyme would provide the optimal molecular approach. Though this has been achieved in the mouse,[66] the porcine stem cells needed for this approach are not yet available.

Concerns have been expressed as to the role of endothelial cell activation in xenograft rejection and research is being carried out into the molecular mechanisms involved. A key transcription factor, NF-κB, which is needed to upregulate the genes involved in endothelial cell activation has now been identified. The action of this factor is naturally inhibited by another factor, IκBα, whose action can be upregulated to prevent NF-κB activation and so reduce the degree of endothelial cell activation.

Tolerance to antigens on a porcine graft that would normally elicit a response by the recipient would prevent the need for long-term immuno-suppression. In xenotransplantation the possibility exists for both donor and recipient manipulation to achieve this. It has been shown possible to achieve T cell tolerance in a pig-to-mouse model and further studies are underway in the pig-to-primate model.[67] More elusive is the goal of B cell tolerance with the aim of removing or inactivating the xenoreactive B cell

215

clones responsible for humoral rejection of a xenograft. Advances in this area could dramatically improve xenograft survival.

Conclusion

Rapid progress has been made in understanding the molecular mechanisms of xenograft rejection. This has allowed the development of successful strategies which prevent hyperacute rejection and short-term survival of transgenic pig xenografts in primate recipients can now consistently be achieved. Before xenotransplantation can be extended into the clinical arena it will be necessary to demonstrate longer term survival with an immunosuppressive regimen that can be safely used in human recipients. The precise definition of what that "longer term" survival should be before human clinical xenotransplantation commences remains a subject of debate. Some workers have suggested that median survivals of "weeks or months" would be an adequate benchmark for likely clinical success[68] whereas others suggest that survival should be equivalent to that seen in comparable allograft models.[69] Whatever the time chosen, even the most exhaustive of research does not provide a guarantee of clinical success and the first clinical xenotransplants will have to be regarded as "clinical experiments". This will undoubtedly attract criticism but demonstration of a reasonable expectation of success and clear explanation of the rationale and a statement of the goals of the xenotransplant itself should allay many concerns.

References

1 Reemtsma K, McCracken BH, Schlegel JU et al. Renal heterotransplantation in man. *Ann Surg* 1964;3:384–410.
2 Reemtsma K, McCracken BH, Schlegel JU et al., Reversal of early graft rejection after renal heterotransplantation in man. *JAMA* 1964;187:691–6.
3 Starzl TE, Marchioro TL, Peters GN et al. Renal heterotransplantation from baboon to man: experience with six cases. *Transplantation* 1964;2:752–76.
4 Caine N, O'Brien V. Quality of life and psychological aspects of heart transplantation. In: Wallwork J. Ed. *Heart and heart-lung transplantation*. Philadelphia: WB Saunders, 1989.
5 Caine N, Sharples L, English TAH, Wallwork J. Prospective study comparing quality of life before and after heart transplantation. *Transplant Proc* 1990;22:1437–9.
6 Cooley DA, Hallman GL, Bloodwell RD, Nora JJ, Leachman RD. Human Heart Transplantation, experience with twelve cases. *Am J Cardiol* 1968;22:804–10.
7 Chen JM, Michler RE. Heart xenotransplantation: lessons learned and future prospects. *J Heart Lung Transplant* 1993;12:869–75.
8 Barnard CN., Wolpowitz A, Losman JG. Heterotopic cardiac transplantation with a zenograft for assistance of the left heart in cardiogenic shock after cardiopulmonary bypass. *S Afr Med J* 1977;52:1035–8.
9 Bailey LL., Nehlsen-Cannarella SL., Concepcion W, Jolley WB. Baboon-to-human cardiac xenotransplantation in a neonate. *JAMA* 1985;254:3321–9.
10 Czaplicki J, Blonska B, Religa Z. The lack of hyperacute xenogeneic heart rejection in a human. *J Heart Lung Transplant* 1992;11:393–6.

11 Gore S. The shortage of donor organs: whither, not whether. *Xeno* 1993;1:23–4.
12 Calne RY. Organ transplantation between widely disparate species. *Transplant Proc* 1970;2:550–3.
13 Hammer, C. Evolutionary physiological and immunological consideration in defining a suitable donor for man. In: Cooper DKC, Kemp E, Reemtsma K, White DJG. eds. *Xenotransplantation. The transplantation of organs and tissues between species.* Berlin: Springer-Verlag, 1991.
14 Platt JL, Lindman BJ, Chen, H, Spitalnik SL, Bach, FH. Endothelial cell antigens recognized by xenoreactive human natural antibodies. *Transplantation* 1990;50:817–22.
15 Good AH, Cooper DKC, Malcolm AJ et al. Identification of carbohydrate structures that bind human anti-porcine antibodies: implications for discordant xenografting in humans. *Transplant Proc* 1992;24:559.
16 Galili U., Kobrin E, Shohet SB, Stults CLM, Macher BA. Man, apes and other old world monkeys differ from other animals in the expression of α-galactosyl epitopes on nucleated cells. *J Biol Chem* 1988;263:17755–62.
17 Larsen RD, Rivera-Marrero CA, Ernst LK, Cummings RD, Lowe JD. Frameshift and nonsense mutations in a human genomic sequence homologous to a murine UDP-Galβ-D-Gal(1,4)-D-GlcNAcα(1,3) galactosyltransferase cDNA. *J Biol Chem* 1990;265:7055–62.
18 Galili U, Swanson K. Gene sequences suggest inactivation of α1-3 galactosyltransferase in catarrhines after the divergence of apes from monkeys. *Proc Natl Acad Sci USA* 1991;88:7401–4.
19 Vanhove B, Bach FH. Human xenoreactive natural antibodies – avidity and targets on porcine endothelial cells. *Transplantation* 1993;56:1251–3.
20 Galili U, Rachmilewitz EA, Peleg A, Flechner I. A unique natural human antibody with anti-α-galactosyl specificity. *J Exp Med* 1984;160:1519–31.
21 Galili U, Mandrell RE, Hamadeh RA, Shohet SB, Griffiss JMcL. Interaction between human natural anti-α-galactosyl immunoglobulin G and bacteria of the human flora. *Infect Immun* 1988;56:1730–7.
22 Kujundzic KM, Koren E, Neethling FA et al. Variability of anti-αGal antibodies in human serum and their relation to serumcytotoxicity against pig cells. *Xenotransplantation* 1994;1:58–65.
23 Casali P, Notkins AL. CD5+ B lymphocytes, polyreactive antibodies and the human B-cell repertoire. *Immunol Today* 1989;10:364–8.
24 Gonzales R, Charlemagne J, Mahana W, Avrameas S. Specificity of natural serum antibodies present in phylogenetically distinct fish species. *Immunology* 1988;63:31–6.
25 Adachi H, Rosengard BR, Hutchins GM, et al. Effects of cyclosporine, aspirin and cobra venom factor on discordant cardiac xenograft survival in rats. *Transplant Proc* 1987;19:1145–8.
26 Leventhal JR, Dalmasso AP, Cromwell JW et al. Prolongation of cardiac xenograft survival by depletion of complement. *Transplantation* 1993;55:857–66.
27 Zhow X-J, Nielson N, Pawlowski I et al. Prolongation of survival of discordant kidney xenografts by C6 deficiency. *Transplantation* 1990;50:896–8.
28 Miyagawa S, Hirose H, Shirakura R et al. The mechanism of discordant xenograft rejection. *Transplantation* 1988;46:825–30.
29 Johnston PS, Wang M-W, Lim SML, Wright LJ, White DJG. Discordant xenograft rejection in an antibody-free model. *Transplantation* 1992;54:573–6.
30 Platt JL, Dalmasso AP, Lindman BJ, Ihrcke NS, Bach FH. The role of C5a and antibody in the release of heparan sulphate from endothelial cells. *Eur J Immunol* 1991;21:2887.
31 Vercellotti GM, Platt JL, Bach FH, Dalmasso AP. Neutrophil adhesion to xenogeneic endothelium through iC3b. *J Immunol* 1991;146:730–4.
32 Pober, JS, Cotran RS. Cytokines and endothelial cell biology. *Physiol Rev* 1990;70:427–51.
33 Vanhove B, Bach FH. Human xenoreactive natural antibodies: avidity and targets on porcine endothelial cells. *Transplantation* 1993;56:1251–3.
34 Platt JL, Vercellotti GM, Lindman B. et al. Release of heparan sulfate from endothelial cells. *J Exp Med* 1990;171:1363–8.
35 Pober, JS, Cotran RS. The role of endothelial cells in inflammation. *Transplantation* 1990;50:537–44.

36 Platt JL, Holzknecht ZE. Porcine platelet antigens recognised by human xenoreactive natural antibodies. *Tansplantation* 1994;57:327–35.
37 Lumpugnani MG, Resnati M, Dejana E, Marchisio PC. The role of integrins in the maintenance of endothelial cell monolayer integrity. *J Cell Biol* 1991;112:479.
38 Saadi S, Platt JL. Transient perturbation of endothelial integrity induced by natural antibody and complement. *J Exp Med* 1995;181:21–31.
39 Hammer C, Chaussy C, von Scheel J, *et al.* Survival times of skin and kidney grafts within different canine species in relation to their genetic markers. *Transplant Proc* 1975;7:439–47.
40 Lim SML, White DJG. Both concordant and discordant heart xenografts are rejected by athymic (nude) rats with same tempo as in T cell competent animals. *Transplant Proc* 1991;23:581–3.
41 Thomas FT, Marchman W, Carobbi A *et al.* Immunobiology of the xenograft response: xenograft rejection in immunodeficient animals. *Transplant Proc* 1991;23:208–9.
42 Van den Bogaerde JB, Aspinall R, Wang M-W *et al.* Induction of long-term survival of hamster heart xenografts in rats. *Transplantation* 1991;52:15–20.
43 Steinbruchel DA, Nielsen B, Salomon S, Kemp E. Sequential, morphological and anti-donor antibody analysis in a hamster-to-rat heart transplantation model. *Transplant Int* 1992;5:38–42.
44 Van den Bogaerde J, Aspinall R, Wang M-W *et al.* Induction of long-term survival of hamster heart xenografts in rats. *Transplantation* 1991;52:15–20.
45 Moses RD, Pierson RN, III, Winn HJ, Auchincloss H Jr. Xenogeneic proliferative and helper lymphokine production are dependent on CD4+ helper cells and self antigen-presenting cells in the mouse. *J Exp Med* 1990;172:567–75.
46 Pierson RN III, Winn HJ, Russell PS, Auchincloss H Jr. Xenogeneic skin graft rejection is especially dependent on CD4+ T cells. *J Exp Med* 1989;170:991–6.
47 Auchincloss H Jr. Why is cell-mediated xenograft rejection so strong? *Xeno* 1995;3:19–22.
48 Kirk AD, Li RA, Kinch MS *et al.* The humanantiporcine cellular repertoire: in vitro studies of acquired and innate cellular responsiveness. *Transplantation* 1993;55:924–31.
49 Reding R, Davies HffS, White DJG. *et al.* Effect of plasma exchange on guinea-pig to rat heart xenografts. *Transplant Proc* 1989;21:534–6.
50 Van de Stadt J, Vendeville B, Wiell B. *et al.* Discordant heart xenografts in the rat. *Transplantation* 1988;45:514–18.
51 Fischel RJ, Matas AJ, Platt JL *et al.* Cardiac xenografting in the pig-to-rhesus monkey model: manipulation of antiendothelial antibody prolongs survival. *J Heart Lung Transplant* 1992;11:965–74.
52 Hasan R, van den Bogaerde JB, Wallwork J, White DJG. Evidence that long term survival of concordant xenografts is achieved by inhibition of antispecies antibody production. *Transplantation* 1992;54:408–13.
53 Murase N, Starzl TE, Demetris AJ *et al.* Hamster-to-rat heart and liver xenotransplantation with FK506 plus antiproliferative drugs. *Transplantation* 1993;55:701–8.
54 Pruitt SK, Baldwin WM III, Marsh HC Jr, *et al.* The effect of soluble complement receptor type 1 on hyperacute xenograft rejection. *Transplantation* 1991;52:868–73.
55 Pruitt SK, Kirk AD, Bollinger RR *et al.* The effect of soluble complement receptor type 1 on hyperacute rejection of porcine xenografts. *Transplantation* 1994;57:363–70.
56 Atkinson JP, Farries T. Separation of self from non-self in the complement system. *Immunol Today* 1987;8:212–15.
57 Oglesby TJ, White DJG, Tedja I *et al.* Protection of mammalian cells from complement-mediated lysis by transfection of human membrane cofactor protein (MCP) and decay accelerating factor (DAF). *Trans Assoc Am Phys* 1991;104:164.
58 Oglesby TJ, Allen CJ, Liszewski MK, White DJG, and Atkinson JP. Membrane cofactor protein (CD46) protects cells from complement-mediated attack by an intrinsic mechanism. *J Exp Med* 1992;175:1547–51.
59 McCurry KR, Kooyman DL, Alvarado CG *et al.* Human complement regulatory proteins protect swine-to-primate cardiac xenografts from humoral injury. *Nature Med* 1995;1:423–7.

60 Cary N, Moody J, Yannoutsos N, Wallwork J, White DJG. Tissue expression of human decay accelerating factor, a regulator of complement activation expressed in mice: a potential approach to inhibition of hyperacute xenograft rejection. *Transplant Proc* 1993;**25**:400–1.
61 Langford GA, Yannoutsos N, Cozzi E *et al.* Production of pigs transgenic for human decay accelerating factor. *Transplant Proc* 1994;**26**:1400–1.
62 Rosengard, AM, Cary NrB, Langford GA *et al.* Tissue expression of human complement inhibitor, decay-accelerating factor, in transgenic pigs. *Transplantation* 1995;**59**:1325–33.
63 Cozzi E, Langford GA, Richards A *et al.* Expression of human decay accelerating factor in transgenic pigs. *Transplant Proc* 1994;**26**:1402–3.
64 Carrington CA, Richards AC, Cozzi *et al.* Expression of human DAF and MCP on pig endothelial cells protects from human complement. *Transplant Proc* 1995;**27**:321–3.
65 Dunning JJ, Braidley PC, Cozzi E *et al.* Pig hearts transgenic for human decay accelerating factor are protected from hyperacute rejection in primate recipients (abstract). *J Heart Lung Transplant* 1996;**15**:S100.
66 Tearle RG, Tange MJ, Zannettino ZL. The al-3 galactosyltransferase knockout mouse: implications for xenotransplantation. *Transplantation* 1996;**61**:13–19.
67 Sachs DH, Sablinski T. Tolerance across discordant xenogeneic barriers. *Xenotransplantation* 1995;**2**:234–9.
68 Pierson RN III, White DJG, Wallwork J. Ethical considerations in clinical cardiac xenografting. *J Heart Lung Transplant* 1993;**12**:876–8.
69 Steele DKR, Auchincloss H Jr. Xenotransplantation. *Annu Rev Med* 1995;**46**:345–60.
70 Hardy JD, Chavez CM, Kurrus FD *et al.* Heart transplantation in man: developmental studies and report of a case. *JAMA* 1964;**188**:114–22.

INDEX

221

fluid management, organ donors 38–9, 50
folinic acid 137
fungal infections 86, 87
  antifungal resistance 88
  in lung recipients 177, 178, 179
  myocardial pathology 106
  patient lifestyle and 88–9
  prophylaxis 177
  pulmonary histopathology 116

ganciclovir
  prophylactic 83, 84, 137, 176–7
  therapy 83–4
gastrointestinal infections 86–7
gout 138

health insurance 19
heart
  donor
    matching to recipient 51
    "oversized", in pulmonary
      hypertension 6
    removal 51–2
  pathology of excised 934
  total artificial 10, 12
heart disease
  contraindicating lung transplant
    16–17, 161
  indicating heart transplant 3–4, 9,
    48–9
heart donors
  management 50–1
  shortage 60
  suitability criteria 38, 50–1
heart failure *see* cardiac failure
heart-lung transplantation (HLT)
  history 156–7
  indications 6, 16, 17, 62–3, 64,
    161–3
  operative procedure 68–9, 70
  survival 21
heart rate, heart recipients 53, 145
heart rejection
  acute *see* acute heart rejection
  chronic 116–18 *see also* coronary
    artery disease, graft
  hyperacute 56
heart transplantation
  cardiac complications 145–53
  histopathology 93–127
  history 48
  long-term management 132–43

mechanical circulatory support
  before 10–13
  numbers 1–2
  operation 51–5
  perioperative complications 56–60
  repeat 12–13, 150
  selection of patients 1–13, 48–9
  waiting period 49–50
  xenogeneic 195–6
height, matching for 51
hepatic disease
  as contraindication 6, 16, 160
  pulmonary hypertension with 25
hepatitis 6
hepatitis B infection 7, 17, 80
hepatitis C infection 17, 80
herpes simplex infections 83, 87, 116
  prophylaxis 176
  therapy 137
  v cytomegalovirus infections 124
herpes zoster (shingles) 87, 137
heterotopic heart transplantation
  operative procedure 52–3, 55
  xenogeneic 195–6
histopathology 93–127
HLA
  disparity, role in rejection 118
  matching 51
HMG CoA reductase inhibitors
  (statins) 138, 152
"hormone cocktail", organ donors 45
hormone replacement therapy 141
hospital-acquired (nosocomial)
  infections 59, 82–3, 90
human immunodeficiency virus (HIV)
  infection 7, 17, 80
humoral immunity *see also* antibodies
  in heart rejection 97, 118
hyperacute heart rejection 56
hyperacute xenograft rejection 200–5
  complement system 202–4
  endothelium and 204–5
  histopathology 200
  preformed xenoreactive antibodies
    201–2
  strategies to prevent 208–9
  target antigens 200–1
hyperlipidaemia 138, 152
hypertension 18
  in heart recipients 58, 137–8, 150
  in severe brain injury 34–5, 39
hypoplastic left heart syndrome 5, 196

225